C000142320

Exercise Is Bad for You

A Short Guide on Being a Better Human

Tyler Thoms, M.S., CSCS

ISBN: 9798645544539

DEDICATION

This book is dedicated to my family, friends, colleagues, clients, mentors, and former students. Thanks for putting up with me. Without you, I never would have been inspired to put it all down on paper. A part of each of you is in every word. From the bottom of my heart, thank you.

Table of Contents

Random blank pages for no reason at all.

I sincerely apologize. I don't know why they're necessary...

Intro

Why are we here? Truth be told, I have no idea. Nor will this book answer that for you, but it got your attention didn't it? Good. First and foremost, thank you for buying this book and investing in yourself. I am not sure if this is actually a book or more of a guide. Regardless, when I began to write it, I intended for it to be more of a guide. A compass, if you will. It is pretty safe to say that you are reading this because you care to improve your health and exercise habits and perhaps need some greater insight as to how to effectively do that. It was at this same point (one random day in the year 2013) where I began my health and fitness journey as well. I was (and still am) very curious how to best approach going about exercise. I knew it was "good for me." but how should I go about it, and what should I prioritize? What is most important? And why the frick did I call my book "Exercise Is Bad For You"? We'll get to that.

Since then, I have earned a bachelors and a masters in the subject and (amongst other things) been a personal trainer and strength coach for roughly 4 years. While this is (relatively) not a long time, I have worked with people of nearly all ages and abilities. It does not take long to spot the good movers (natural athletes) and the bad ones. Most of my clients were just regular people trying to be healthier, not dedicated athletes. Being a personal trainer, I believe that everyone should have (a very skilled and educated) one in their corner. I would even hire one! People should be educated about the one and only body they will ever get. Despite a relatively extensive formal education and a handful of experience, I am still humbled every day as I continue to learn about the human body and how to best treat it. Given the relative cost of skilled practitioners, I hope this guide serves as an alternative (and much cheaper) solution to some of your exercise woes. And believe me, you have woes. We all do, and it's perfectly human to have them. I hope it will at least provide you with a much greater sense of what you should be prioritizing when you exercise and workout. The truth is, there is no one approach that works for all. No matter how bad we want there to be, no one program or diet can fix every health problem you may have. In fact, part of the problem is that there are a great many programs and diets that cause more problems than they solve. I have spent much of my short career trying to find the answers the human body is looking for. I believe there is one direction we should all be heading. The available pathways in that direction are many. Even when pointed in the "right" direction, there are certainly many ways to get things wrong when it comes to your health (obvious ones: not exercising at all, not eating well, etc.) Some of the not so obvious ones, I will discuss within this book. The main purpose of this book is to guide and educate. This relatively short read comprises what I believe to be the most important aspects of training and health; most of which 95% percent of the world's population either doesn't know about or is ignoring.

No matter what form of exercise you choose at any given point in your life, and regardless of gender, I believe these aspects will always hold true for humans. Mind you, this is not an exhaustive list. It is not a guide on how to become a better athlete. It is more so a guide on how to exercise to optimize the human body for what it really is. I certainly do not know everything there is to know about the human body. But I believe I know enough about what is actually important to offer this information to you in a relatively small and easy to digest package. I have found that education is not about changing how smart you are, but more so, how aware you are. I believe regular exercise to be one of the most important factors in good health and happiness. Without your health, it's hard to have much of anything else in this life. I hope to leave you more aware about what is truly important when it comes to that practice. And it is very much a practice. Certainly, exercising is a choice and an investment in more forms than one. It is a physically demanding, long-term endeavor. I find myself always mentioning to clients that "it's a marathon, not a sprint". So, it is important to find activities/programs that are enjoyable and motivating for the long term. Let this be "point number one" that I want to make. Rest assured, nothing in this guide will mean anything to you if you are not choosing to consistently and seriously pursue your health through the practices mentioned herein. Let's be clear that one thing that will always hold true with regards to your health, is that you must pursue it. It will not happen by chance or accident. It must be consistent, progressive, and long-term to experience any meaningful benefits. However, this book does not explore the various programs, trends and/or fads that are available to us. For one, there are way too many to mention. Secondly, given that they are ever-changing, this book would quickly become obsolete if I discussed topics that only held true for a few months. Perhaps, that type of information might be better suited for an article in a magazine. The thing with exercise is, much like fashion, it is surrounded by a great deal of trends and fads that are constantly changing and evolving alongside what is "in". You do not have to be an expert in this field (or fashion for that matter) to realize this. You simply have to be willing to pay attention. From Cross Fit, Zumba, Pilates, Hot Yoga, club sports, or other various group and individual exercise programs, there are a myriad of different options to choose from. All of them claim to be "the best". The same goes for the insane amount of diet programs we have at our disposal. For the record, I think all programs and diets have their respective weaknesses. Some of them have weaknesses that are more glaring than others. But I will not get into that here. If anything, no matter what program/method you subscribe to, I just hope for your sake that it takes into account the topics that I will discuss and that you subscribe to the one that works best for you. So, what do we do with all these options? I suppose the best option is to try one out and see if you like it. Maybe you don't choose any of them and instead walk the road alone. You go to the gym by yourself 2-3 times a week with no real idea what you are doing and hope that what you are doing is beneficial in both the short and long term. Here is the issue. This is why I chose to compose this book. There are too many trends, fads, and programs. There are too many trainers/gyms/brands pushing their "unique" product or exercises on every available platform known to man to make a quick buck or just to get you to hit that ever important "like" button. And I'll be blunt, I think most of them are crap. You might think to yourself "hey, isn't that what YOU are doing right now? Pushing a product?" Yes. However, I am not pushing information that I claim to be new or unique. I am not creating another trend or brand. I am simply offering this guide in an attempt to re-focus our approach using information (that most of us either don't know about or that we ignore) that has been around for a long time (i.e. not crap). I believe the answers to a happy and healthy body are already out there. Many of us just need help navigating all the aforementioned crap. There are good and meaningful trends in health and fitness. There is a ton of relevant and accurate information already available to us. But it is eclipsed by the mass of fitness trends/fads that seem to make it onto our social media pages more often than not. I hope to uncover some of these truths for you via this book.

Speaking of endless exercise options, you know what can happen when people have way too many options to choose from? They choose not to choose. They become discouraged, confused, and then give up for fear that what they choose won't be the best for them. Either that, or they continue on their current path doing what is "in". It goes something like: "I saw that guy doing it and he was really fit, so I think I'll do it too and hope for the same results." Sound familiar at all? There is too much of that going on and if we are honest with ourselves, we are all guilty of it at one point or another. This type of approach leads to varied results, some of which include a great deal of injury and pain. And what does injury and pain lead to? More discouraged and confused people that give up on their health. It results in a great deal of people blaming the activities/programs themselves instead of questioning the process, methodology, or even their own choices. People are so confused and misled. If you look close enough, you can see it in the way they move. You can see it in their daily habits. Just days after writing this passage, I saw a dad and his son (the boy was somewhere near 10 or 11 years old) working out in the gym while I was with a client. Before doing some sort of deadlift variation with dumbbells, he asked his son "How much do you weigh?" Now having both his son's and my own attention. I was confused why this boy's father needed to know his weight in the middle of a workout. His son answered with "About 127." His dad looks up in the air as if he's deep in thought and he says "Okay, 75% of that, so, grab two 35's". My thoughts: First of all, why are you basing the weight he should use for the impending exercise on just his body weight? Secondly, why is 75% the magical number? And third, 75% of 127 is about 95lbs...Two 35's is 70 lbs...*Just what in the heck was I witnessing here?* Long story short, the poor kid didn't come even close to getting the dumbbells off of the ground, let alone lifting them with any sort of form that might be considered safe. I can only imagine these types of shenanigans are not uncommon elsewhere.

We are past due for change. Unfortunately for us all, there is a crazy amount of misinformation floating around this industry. There is an insane amount of deception and it almost always revolving around money. Gyms all around the world share a business model that profits on the hope that you will sign up, pay your monthly dues, and then never come again. Every trainer in those gyms thinks they know best. How can I prove that I actually know best? I can't. Again, nor do I think I know everything. But something has gone awry. I can smell it in the air. I just believe I know enough to sound the alarms. These aspects of health/exercise are not ones I believe will change much over time. I unapologetically state that much of the following information will always hold true inside my mind. It will hold true as long as we still call ourselves humans. It will hold true no matter how big, small, wide, thin, tall, short, heavy, light, strong, or weak you find yourself throughout your life. Many of these points are "human trends" that, whether we like it or not, will never change. Mind you, much of this is based on my education and exposure to loads of research on various exercise science topics. Some of it is based on my opinion and my overall take on the relatively small body of knowledge that sits within my brain. It is not the answer to everything related to exercise. I wrote this book because this information needs to be heard. My intent is to educate and help my readers in finding their path. When it comes to your body, ignorance is not bliss. This book is an opinion piece from me to you. It is a book for both you and I. Why is it a book for me? This book also serves to relieve a great deal of frustration regarding where the exercise industry is currently at. Some of the ways some industry "professionals" make money off of consumers should be a crime. Instagram trainers are loading their pages with exercise ideas/demonstrations/methods that they say everyone should be doing. Why should everyone do it? Usually, because it gets them more followers and makes them more money. Some may play a part in the cause of your pain/dysfunction either now or in the future. One of the first and most important points I'd like to make now is that just because something doesn't cause you pain now, does not mean it isn't bad for you in the long term. Many of the ideas these influential figures promote are temporary "quick fixes"; proverbial band-aids. If they were to be honest, these influencers know they are handing out band-aids too. They keep you coming back for more to keep them in business.

Got back pain? Great, no problem. Here is a 60 second video that will do just the trick! I'm sorry, but the human body is just not that simple and making people think that is just lazy. Again, I have mentioned that all of this exercise stuff was a long-term investment. We should all be careful where we hedge our bets. Spend too much time in the wrong market and you might end up broke(n). You only get one body that thrives for somewhere around 20-25 years. After that, it's downhill. It's downhill no matter what. Should we not do our best to apply the brakes and slow that descent the best we can?

After you read this relatively short book (hopefully in its entirety), it is up to you to decide what path you will continue on. My one and only goal in writing is to leave you more aware. While the content areas are broad, the scope of this book is really quite small. I hope it serves as a simple means of getting you on the right track and keeping you there with minimal regard to the infinite number of other details and outside influences associated with your health. It's basically "how to be a better human" in about 100 pages. Once again, I liken it to a compass. You may stray from your current path many times. You may be pulled away from any one given thing at any time. Regardless, I hope the information found here will keep you pointed in the "right direction" at all times, throughout your entire life. The topics that follow are aspects of training/exercising/working out (whatever you want to call it) that we all need to be, at the very least, made aware of. Basically, these are the things that I have always wished I could tell everyone I meet who engages in regular exercise. Some of the points I offer are just general information. For others, I offer what (I think) you should or should not do. Regardless, I do not intend to convince you that what you are doing or will do is right or wrong. For what it's worth, I hope this information serves to open your mind and focus it upon the pieces of the exercise/health equation that I find to be most important based on my experience and education.

There is a great deal of deception in this industry and things are much too complicated. It is an understatement to say that it all bothers me. It bothers me because many of us blindly follow somebody else's lead without asking why; without making the choice to educate ourselves before acting. With all of this misinformation floating around, the fitness industry (which is almost entirely unregulated by the way) is in a very dark place. The masses are ignorant and look to exercise professionals to lead them. As a whole, we are failing them. If we are not already there, I believe we have been and are still spiraling toward a human population ridden with dysfunction and pain. No matter the scale, I hope this book is revered by readers as an attempt at shining light upon the real truths regarding the human body. Myths will be debunked; egos will be shattered. Brace yourself for a call for change in the form of a book that goes against the grain of today's fitness industry as we know it.

Just trying to lengthen the book at this point...

1

Everybody's the Same at Being Different

Okay, here we go. Let's begin with a few overarching themes. One of the most important things to remember about humans is that we all develop and move similarly, yet individual differences will always exist. That is as complicated as it really needs to be for the sake of this book. During the time of writing this book, I was teaching a course on motor development at California State University, Bakersfield. This was one of the overarching themes of the course and something that is important to realize when approaching exercise habits. We might move and develop in many similar ways, but what works for you won't necessarily work for others. The way you perform exercises may look different than the way I do. This does not necessarily mean mine are better quality than yours. Everyone has different levels of fitness, athleticism, coordination, self-esteem, motivation, sociocultural influences, etc.. I won't get into all of these developmental factors that might have an effect on your movement. However, when you really dive into them, you realize it becomes really hard to compare yourself to others with any real accuracy. This is generally why I have a huge problem with Instagram/Facebook pages constantly posting exercises that "you should be doing". Right, nothing is better than hundreds of thousands (maybe more) of followers doing the same exact exercise, the same exact way the super fit guy is doing it on his 60-second video. Thanks fitness "professional". And we wonder why our society is more and more ridden with pain/injury.

Due to physical and physiological variability amongst the population, assessment of your individual fitness level is important before beginning a program/routine. This can give you a good idea where to start or how to continue your journey to make sure you are always progressing. If you aren't consistently progressing, you might maintain certain aspects of fitness, but you certainly will not become more fit. Regardless of where you are in your own journey, one thing is for sure: you must take an individualized approach, and it must progress (essentially, become more difficult) regularly. By the way, I am not a fan of the term "exercise routine" for these reasons. Routine makes it sound like you do the same thing over and over again, day after day, year after year. This is certainly not what I am preaching. Exercise should be a routine. How you exercise should not become routine for long. This is where adaptation and progression toward higher levels of fitness stops.

Because exercising requires an individualized approach, it is my opinion that comparing yourself to others should be minimized. Exercise for you. Pay attention to your journey. Compare yourself to where you were weeks, months, or years ago and I'll bet you find more results, longer-lasting motivation, and less discouragement. Also be aware that everyone will respond to the same exercise stimulus in different ways. Let this be one of the overarching themes within this book. Many people will read research or read an article, "copy and paste" it into their life and either not get the results that were advertised, injure themselves, or both. Some may get the results they sought, but not everyone. This is normal. While it is definitely important to consider, much of the research on the human body is both flawed and inconclusive. There are certainly reliable trends, but almost never material that can be considered absolutely concrete. It is important that you take all reliable information at hand into consideration, and then tweak it to suit your body and your needs. Due to our variability, you may see exercise recommendations, but you will not see any set or repetition recommendations within this book. Nor will you find a "one of a kind" exercise program written by yours truly guaranteed to get you results. Promising you amazing results after having read this book would be careless. Pointing you in the right direction or providing you with a place to start your approach, however, is much more honorable in my book (no pun intended). Let's dive in.

2

Everything is Connected to Everything

This is something not many people are aware of. All systems of the body are connected and play off of one another. Exactly how each of these systems connect and how much one influences the other is beyond my knowledge and the scope of this book. However, there is a growing body of research on these topics. A different (and much longer) book could be written on this topic alone. However, I still feel it is very important to note. In nearly all of the textbooks I have read throughout my high school and college experiences, they break up each system into individual chapters so that it is easier to learn and mentally digest. You learn about the nervous system, then the digestive, endocrine, and so on. I cannot recall a single textbook that mentioned that all of these systems are in some way connected to one another. Needless to say, it gets very complex and I am not about to dive into all of it (you're welcome). I will offer a few pieces of information though to at least give you some idea.

The brain is king. The brain has the first and final say of everything that goes on inside your body. Jeff Hawkins is the creator of the Palm Pilot and one of the leading researchers in neuroscience today. According to Jeff's research, the brain operates under the direction and influence of sensory & motor patterns and various predictions. The brain has trillions of various types of nerves that carry and store information received from the body throughout your entire life. The brain is also responsible for sending out information to the body, such as when we initiate movement. There is a constant flow of information and the brain is always keeping a tab on what is going on with your body and all of the systems inside it. Basically, it is the best security guard of all time. Nothing gets past it or goes on with its say so. Does it make errors? Sure, a lot. But it remembers and learns from them. The brain is like a computer, except that it has the amazing ability to store information and then subsequently make intelligent and accurate predictions based on both stored information as well as information it is constantly receiving. There is no computer like it. Whereas computers operate strictly based on their installed software/operating systems; brains are malleable. To learn more about your brain in much greater (and more eloquent) detail, I suggest buying the book "On Intelligence" written by Jeff Hawkins himself. It will blow your mind (pun-intended). We will talk more about the importance of the brain and how it pertains to exercise later on. However, the main point is this: The brain receives all information and is the most advanced organ in the body. However, as amazing as it is, it is fairly easy to trick and makes a ton of mistakes.

Ever wonder why we get carsick? This is because the visual (eyes) and vestibular (balance) systems are intimately connected. After all, they sit right next to each other inside our skulls. It is not that surprising. When you look down in the car, your visual system sends a signal to your brain telling it "you are in a stable environment". However, in walks the vestibular system and it says, "wait just one hot second, partner, we are not in a stable environment. My sources tell me we are moving quite fast. In fact, there's lots of speeding up and slowing down". I don't know why the vestibular system sounds like it's from the wild west. But the brain receives these conflicting messages and says "Uh oh. Time to call on the enteric nervous system to fix this." Turns out the enteric nervous system is kind of a jerk in this situation and says, "time for the visual system to see previously-ingested food again." And boom. We find some "relief" as well as quite an unpleasant mess. Here, we see the brain is easily tricked and actually quite terrible at problem solving. "Problem? Okay, must be the food. Make human throw up now. All better." Luckily, our brain is intelligent in the way that it stores this memory for later use. This later use comes in the form of the thought "hey, maybe I should NOT look down for long periods of time while in a fast-moving vehicle". Thus, we have progress. This is just one example of how two or more systems might connect. Stay tuned for more.

3

Exercise Is Bad For You

Let's get one thing straight right off the bat here: exercise is bad for you. Wait, what? Yes. It's bad. Going for a nice, long run puts stress on all systems of your body (yes, including your immune system). Depending on how much you weigh and how fast you run, each step sends roughly 4-5 times your body weight through your knee joint, into your hip and up the chain. Even your jawbone accepts some of this force. Exercise increases activity within the sympathetic nervous system. Simply put, it's stressful. It activates the "fight or flight" response within your brain. The same response that our brains interpret as feeling we are in danger. We stop digesting, our heart rate increases, we sweat, we smell, and, after an amount of time, we feel fatigued. A lot of the time, we are fatigued for the next several days. Why? Because it's bad. That's why. When you repetitively lift heavy weights, you are literally tearing muscle fibers within those targeted muscle groups (that is what soreness is). You are depleting your body of stored energy. You are tiring your brain. You are damaging yourself. Your body does not like it. It is no wonder so many people hate exercise. It's almost entirely a negative experience for the human. Each and every time you workout. Yay.

I know what you might be thinking. "Gee golly, what a great way to start the book, dude." Before you put it down, be aware that this negative experience, this damage, is absolutely necessary for the most important part! Rest and recovery. Unfortunately, we have to break ourselves down to build ourselves back up. This is the first and one of the most important points I will make. Exercise is bad, but it is undeniably the most crucial precursor and stimulus for growth and development during the rest period that follows. The benefits that come from this "damage" are nearly endless. Why aren't more of us doing it? Oh right, because it's bad and it sucks. This is the very important point here, folks. It is not the exercise that is good for you. It is the rest and recovery afterwards that is good for you. It is insanely important that you take time off from training to allow your body to rest and rebuild itself stronger than it was before you broke it down. This includes taking care of your diet and sleep habits. I cannot say this enough: your diet, sleep quantity, and sleep quality is paramount in your rest periods. What is a rest period? For the sake of this guide, it is anytime you are not exercising, but it is even more complicated than that. We will get there. The better your rest, the better your recovery and subsequent bouts of exercise. The better your exercise, the greater the stimulus you create for adaptation and improvement. It's easy. Okay, not really.

Routinely Remodeling Routines

An hour is not enough. An hour of exercise in a 24-hour day is not enough. An hour a day three times a week is not enough. Our bodies need more movement than this. We need consistently different types of movement. We need more movement in different places, at different times of the day. We need variability in our movement habits. Many of us attend the gym and fall into a "routine." While this is comforting because it is predictable and gets easier and easier to follow, it is not enough and eventually our bodies and brains will shrug off this activity and adaptation will cease. We all know what it feels like to get bored. Nothing sounds fun. You want to do something, yet at the same time you kind of don't, and you just want to sit there and eat an entire carton of Dreyer's slow-churned ice cream (cookies & cream is my favorite). The brain and body do this too. Except they get bored at the physiological and mechanical levels. Doing the same thing over and over will make your brain bored, so much so that the demand for adaptation significantly decreases. Variability in the amount of time we exercise, when we exercise (time of day), where we exercise (the environment), and what we do while we are exercising (the movements themselves) are all extremely important. If you are at all able to, it is important that we all vary these aspects of our "routine," consistently. This keeps the brain's interest. It can be as simple as trying this out for a week: break away from the gym, and make a promise to yourself that you're going to exercise in a few different environments, at different times of the day, for a varying amount of time, utilizing various movements each day, four times a week, and then see how you feel. I'd be amazed if you didn't feel more *alive* .

4

Frequency, Intensity, Time, and Type (The FITT Principle)

Now, don't get the idea that just because I said to rest a lot means that all you should do is rest. You are probably reading this partly due to the alarming amount of time you do find yourself at "rest" (i.e. not exercising). Obviously, resting more often than not is not the point. This is a balancing act. Just like all other aspects of a healthy lifestyle, you need to effectively mix in work (exercise/movement) and rest. Be aware, it takes relatively a lot more time to recover after a workout than it does to damage yourself from it. We have all been there: the one-hour workout that leaves us bed-ridden, unable to walk right for days. All because you saw a post by a popular Instagram trainer that said you should always go hard on leg day. Oh, and "never skip leg day." Blah, blah, blah. The point is, you did an intense hour-long workout, and now it takes anywhere from 24-72 hours to fully recover. Talk about return on investment! Awesome. Here is another point I wish to make. It should never be the goal to be sore the next day. While being sore is not the worst thing to happen due to a workout, it does not necessarily mean you had a good workout or even performed the exercises correctly. It just means you did damage. Yikes. We'll get more into "good workouts" in Chapter 14.

For now, let's talk about frequency, intensity, time, and type. This is referred to in many textbooks as the FITT principle. While this can be found all over the industry, people really mess this one up often. So, I find it to be an important topic. At some point, we have all wondered "how often should I work out? How long? How much? What weight? What program? Can I just go to sleep instead?" ...and so on. How about you ask a trainer? Some people will, some won't. Regardless, any trainer who doesn't start his/her answer with "it depends" is probably not the best in the business. It all depends. The FITT principle is just the tip of the iceberg, but it is an important one. All four of the variables of the FITT principle can be manipulated to achieve an optimal and healthy stimulus for improvement. Long story short, it takes a good amount of experimentation and even more patience to get it right. Since everyone is the same at being different, what works for some won't always work for others as well. The first step in manipulating each of the following variables should be deciding what your short- and long-term goals are. That will help shape your approach.

Frequency

This is how often you work out. Once a week is probably too little, even for beginners or those that are detrained. 6-7 times a week without adequate rest (depending on your fitness level) may prove to be too much. In my experience, once you have some training experience, 3-4 times a week with interspersed rest days is optimal. It is important that you hit what is referred to as the "minimally effective dose." This is the least amount of work you need to do to ensure you achieve the necessary stimulus for adaptation. Essentially, it is the threshold you need to break each time you work out. The more and longer you work out, the higher this threshold goes (the more fit you become). Where is that point for you? Well, it depends on the following:

- What type of exercise do you engage in?
- Relative to your fitness level, how intense are your workouts?

- How long do you work out each time you go?
- Are you somewhat tired after your sessions? Unphased? Exhausted?
- What does the rest of your day look like? Stressful?
- Relaxing? Somewhere in between?
- Have you been working out often or are you just starting out/returning to exercise?

There is no one right answer for everyone here. It is hard to say unless you have found some perfect way to accurately measure everything during your workouts (heart rate, calories burned, sets, reps, etc.). Using a fitness tracker can help but is definitely more of an estimate. Fear not, there is more (hopefully helpful) insight on this very complex "equation" below.

Intensity

This is how hard you are working per workout OR how hard your overall program is. The context here is important. However, the FITT principle generally refers to how hard a given workout is. Never going hard or going hard all the time is never recommended. Mix up intensity based on how you feel and your overall goals. Throw in a workout that kicks your butt 1-2 times a week. Pay attention to how you feel. If you feel tired, you probably are. Being extremely sore is a classic sign that you did too much. Being a little sore the next day or two means you are pretty close to the sweet spot. You DO NOT have to be sore to create a stimulus for adaptation. You DO NOT have to be sore to grow muscle. Read it again. Soreness is not the goal. Side note: there is hardly any evidence that stretching helps with soreness. So, remember, we are going for longevity! Listen to your body and rest often. If I work out hard 3 times a week because I am too sore to do any more than that, versus Joe Schmo who is working out at a moderate intensity 5 times a week, who will get in more work over the span of the year? Who will provide a stimulus for adaptation and improvement more often? Joe freakin' Shmo (assuming his recovery and dietary habits are of high quality). Intensity (both acute and overall) is important.

Intensity can also be fairly accurately measured by measuring your heart rate (HR). There is a very basic protocol for estimating your maximum HR. Take 220 and subtract your age. This is usually pretty close to your max HR. For instance, if you are 30 years old, subtract 30 from 220 (190), and that is your estimated maximum HR value. The closer you get to that value, the harder you are working. If you are interested, look up "heart rate reserve." It is slightly more complicated, but more accurate and effective than simply basing your workouts off of your max HR. If you have no means or interest in measuring your HR, check out the tip below:

A note on *subjectively* measuring intensity: Within the exercise science field, there is a scale called the Rating of Perceived Exertion (RPE) scale. Some versions of the scale range from 1-20 and more simple representations range from 1-10. I like the 1-10 scale and have found it easier to implement with clients. Basically, in terms of intensity, 1 is the easiest thing you have ever done and 10 is an activity or task that is nearly impossible to do for more than 5-10 seconds. Naturally, 5-6 is somewhere in between. My clients have had great results when I have simply told them to make sure their workouts are always at a 7 or 8. Eventually, a workout that was a 7 from three weeks ago might start to feel like a 5. We would then manipulate the intensity accordingly. RPE can pertain to both a single exercise or the overall program/workout.

Examples

Single Exercise/Set: "Okay Jim, I want you to make this set of lunges an 8 out of 10. Go for it!"

Workout: "Jim, how did that feel today? I was hoping we hit a 7 or 8 for today's workout."

Note to trainers: This is a really easy way to find out if you need to up the intensity or not. I have also found most clients will say a higher value than what it really was to avoid making their workouts more difficult! I have had multiple clients that did not break a sweat or increase their breathing rate that said their workout was a 9. Right...Remember, it's your job to know what will be most beneficial and to know when to push your clients. All this, while sticking to rule #1: Do no harm.

Time

As you may have guessed, this is how long you work during each workout. I cannot really tell you how long you should or should not workout. It's safe to say that 5 minutes is probably too little and 3+ hours straight is way too much for us common folk. Once again, everyone has different fitness levels and this book is not really geared towards the elite athlete. One important note that should be made about time is that it is not necessary to always progress this variable to ensure that your overall program is progressive. I would focus on the other three variables more often. Not that I am the prime example, but my workouts never go past 1.5 hours. I don't know who said it, but I heard one time that "if you are in the gym past 1-1.5 hours, you're just trying to make friends." I like that. I'm sorry, but I have things to do and am not lucky (or good looking) enough to work out for a living. If you are there past 1.5 hours and have not become somewhat fatigued, you are either extremely fit, or you need to up the intensity. My guess is the latter. 1.5 hours (tops) and be on your way to something else!

Type

This refers to the kind of workouts you might engage in. This might include cardio (aerobic) activities, weightlifting (anaerobic activity), high-intensity interval training (HIIT), circuit weight training, or maybe yoga. The list goes on and on. Different types of activities stress the body in different ways. In general, longer-term aerobic training stresses the cardiovascular and respiratory systems more so than the muscular system and vice versa for moderate to heavy weightlifting which also (generally) taxes the nervous system. And yes, there are multiple ways to lift weights aerobically too. Once again, the options for exercise are endless. Pick what you like the most and what motivates you to keep at it. If you get bored, don't give up. Find another option. Personally, I'd stay away from yoga and CrossFit. While I believe yoga can be generally beneficial for the mind and spirit, I offer that it is not the most functional of exercise options as a lot of it involves a great deal of "hypermobile" stretching and orienting your body almost entirely around the force of gravity. I offer that this is not the greatest stimulus for the human structure. Thus, it eats away at our function as well. I will get to what I believe our ultimate function is later on in Chapter 12. CrossFit type workouts, while they may be fun and competitive, often feature members of the general population performing Olympic lifts and other very technical, non-functional movements. Many of their workout formats involve participants performing exercises for "as many reps as possible" or until exhaustion. You also do not need to be a fitness professional to own/operate a CrossFit "box." All of these aspects are red flags to me. But to each his own! Find what you like and use your best judgement. More importantly, always remember the fact that you only get one body. Use it wisely. But I digress.

As I mentioned, each aspect of the FITT principle can be manipulated on a scale ranging low to high. It is a balancing act that depends on a myriad of factors unique to each person. It should make sense that frequency, intensity, and time cannot always be high, or you will experience symptoms of burnout (aka overtraining). If I told you to workout at an intensity that was very taxing, 6-7 days a week, for 3 hours at a time, you'd probably wonder where I got my degrees from (or if they were even real degrees). If these variables were all "low," you'd likely get little to no benefit from your exercise regimen. So, I will leave you with some general guidelines:

- When you significantly increase 1-2 variables of the FITT principle, the other(s) must either stay the same or decrease. The opposite generally holds true as well, see below.
- If you decrease 1-2 variables, the other(s) can safely increase. If you increase ALL of them at once, just know that it cannot last. For instance, if I go from working out for 1 hour, twice per week at an overall RPE of 8 to working out for 2 hours, 4 times a week at the same intensity, I would most likely find this is not feasible. It is too much, too soon.

Herein lies my next point:

- An increase in frequency and/or time usually equates to an automatic increase in overall program intensity. We must be careful when manipulating frequency and time.
- Overall intensity should regularly increase. An increase in intensity might mean you will need to temporarily decrease time and/or frequency (i.e. more rest). Remember, no matter your overall recipe for exercise, high quality rest should be a top priority.

In conclusion, humans need to move well, and we need to move often. We will get into the concept of moving "well" in Chapters 12 and 13. We also need to rest well and rest often. The key word that many people just don't often adhere to is "balance." Too many people either rest too much or workout too much. Both have serious consequences. Manipulate the FITT principle to suit your intentions and individual goals. Not only do we need to move often, but we must provide a consistent stimulus that is intense enough to cause our body and brain to want to adapt.

Your workouts must be progressive to continue seeing results. This is the principle of progressive overload. For some, all of this is a ton of detail. So, what is one simple way to ensure you're generally progressing? Leave the gym taxed, but not exhausted. You should feel "used" when you're done (in a good way, not in a weird high-school relationship kind of way. Don't make this weird). A little soreness isn't bad, but it should never be the goal to be extremely sore 1-3 days later. This is how you know you definitely did too much. While there are some acute beneficial physical and physiological responses to exercise, the results most people care about are never instant. Ever. Accept this and be in it for the long-haul. Results will come with persistence, and they will mean that much more knowing the time and effort you invested.

5

Pre-Workout Practices

For the remainder of the book, I will try and list my points in an order that simulates the process of going to the gym. As we know, you don't necessarily have to go to a gym to get in a workout. In my experience however, most people think "gym" when you say "workout." So, for the sake of simplicity, I will be speaking mostly about workouts held within a gym. Mainly because I believe many of us are prioritizing the wrong stuff when inside them. We will start with what you should do prior to working out, then dive into fairly detailed topics on how you should/shouldn't go about your workout, and finish with some "big picture" stuff (kind of like the beginning). Be forewarned, at some point (perhaps on multiple occasions) I will most likely mention something that you're currently doing that I think you should not do. This is very much a "take it or leave it" type of book. Obviously, I hope you "take it." I believe it is nearly impossible to be influential without ruffling a few feathers along the way. I am okay with that. You will soon find out that I care little about what most people currently prioritize while at the gym. Who knows, I just may change your mind about a few things. Let's dive in.

Pre-Workout Dietary Considerations

Nutrition and dietary recommendations really should be left for nutritionists and dieticians. As a trainer, I can safely say we don't study enough about nutrition past carb, protein, fat, and water intake to know enough to make specific dietary recommendations to our clients. I'd be afraid to work with any trainer (without the proper credentials) that was planning my meals and telling me what he/she thinks I should eat. Let me tell you, this happens all the time. Unless you hire a trainer that has one (or more) of those degrees and/or additional training in the subject, it can be quite dangerous for them to make concrete recommendations. Plus, it is largely dependent on your short- and long-term goals. However, I can say that you need energy to workout, what you eat and how much of it definitely matters, and everyone is different in how their body responds to what they eat. Here are a few things that I can safely say based on what I know about pre-workout dietary recommendations:

Carbohydrates

Carbs (a fancy word for complex sugars) are necessary to fuel exercise. Carbohydrate is just another name for sugar. They can be simple or complex in nature. When you ingest them, your body breaks them down, and they enter your bloodstream for use during your daily activities and/or exercise. Any carbohydrates that aren't needed are stored as glycogen or converted to fat. They are stored in the form of "glycogen" in both your muscles and your liver. Your body draws from these stores if/when necessary. For instance, when you sleep, your body draws from these stores to fuel bodily processes. Same story for when you are fasting (have not eaten in several hours). You can survive for a while on stored fat (also broken down into glycogen when needed) stored glycogen. I don't recommend seeing just how long you can survive without eating...but I digress. Mechanisms of this fuel source and how and when it becomes available is outside the scope of this book. However, my point in mentioning it is to say that since you store glycogen, you actually do not need to eat carbs before a workout. However, it is generally recommended that you do because glycogen runs out relatively quickly, depending on how intense your workout is. Many studies show that ingesting carbs before a workout increases performance measures. Many people, including myself, report feeling better/more energized during their workouts when having eaten beforehand. Some just don't like the feeling of exercising on an empty stomach. Is pre-workout carbohydrate ingestion absolutely necessary though? No. It is especially not necessary if you have eaten a meal within the past 3-4 hours.

Not only do you not absolutely need to eat carbs before a workout, but it is actually generally safe to eat absolutely nothing before a workout too. More and more people are engaging in "intermittent fasting" and, in my book (literally) it's a viable option for weight loss. Many people workout and in some cases, spend the great majority of their day in a fasted state and experience positive results. Many people also do not do so well on this type of regimen. Remember, variability. So, my advice is to experiment and do what works best for you. If you do choose to engage in intermittent fasting, ease into it. Do not fast for 18 hours straight on day one. I don't believe you'll be happy with that decision. Just like with anything else, the body needs time to adapt. Allow it to have that time. In general, if you plan to engage in fairly intense exercise for more than 30 minutes, I recommend eating something 1-2 hours before the start of your workout.

Fats

High fat meals are not recommended right before a workout due to the fact that too much fat can cause an upset stomach during exercise. However, I do not believe everyone experiences this. Again, do what works best for you.

A story and lesson on fats: I had a client a couple years ago that just was not losing weight. (We will get into why I think at a certain point that weight isn't all that important) She was working very hard in the gym and supposedly dieting properly given her overall goals. She had a fairly normal health history. All her "numbers" were good. I was checking off all the boxes I could think of in my head. One night, she was mentioning that her diet had very little fat and she just did not understand how she was still not improving losing weight or fat. Long story short, after asking a few open-ended questions, I came to find out that she meant her diet was low in "bad" fats. I brought to her attention that it was very high in "good" fats (almonds, pumpkin seeds, fish, etc.). She thought this was good. And it is. Sort of. One thing about fats (good or bad) is that they are very high in calories (9 kcal/g). Woah woah woah. What is a kcal? Believe it or not, kcal (meaning 1000 calories) is the correct measurement unit. Most likely, the people that create nutrition labels probably knew that saying that an Oreo cookie has 53,000 calories might scare people away from eating Oreos. Thus, it would not sell. There are many other reasons people should be scared of Oreos, but that is not too relevant here. Man, they are *so* good though. Regardless, kcal is actually the correct term scientists and other nerds (such as myself) use when referring to the amount of energy we consume through our diet. No matter how good your good fats are, too much of any macronutrient will still cause weight gain. Weight loss is simple on paper: calories in versus calories out. Even if you eat 5000 kcal worth of chicken and veggies...you still ate 5000 kcal! Thus, body composition is what we are really concerned with. And that is a whole other animal. We will get into that in Chapter 8.

Protein

Protein is generally safe and sometimes recommended to ingest prior to working out. Once again, this largely depends on your goals. There is a growing body of evidence that suggests whey and casein proteins are the best for muscular hypertrophy (growth) when ingested both pre- and post-workout. However, with a normal and balanced diet, supplementation with protein is usually not always necessary. Do I use protein supplements? Sure. But I believe it is best to get your nutrients from real food. There is also a myth that goes around that those wishing to "bulk up" need to ingest more and more protein. "Do you want to bulk up and put on mass? Eat all the protein!!" The truth is the body will convert other substrates (fats and carbs) into protein if it needs it. Protein is more thermally active than carbs or fats as well. This means that it takes more energy for the body to break it down, resulting in higher caloric expenditure. Generally, people who experience higher caloric expenditure tend to lean out more than bulk up. It is becoming more and more common for those that want to bulk up to simply ingest more calories throughout the day.

A quick note: Protein ingestion and its timing relative to your workout is a hot topic in the exercise world. I am referring to the almighty "anabolic window" and the many myths that surround it. Too many people will tell you that you need to ingest protein immediately after a workout. Like ASAP. "You only have 20-30 minutes, bro. You're gonna lose all your gains if you don't get that shake in you! (*Arnold voice*) Get to the blendaaaa!!" Despite this "enthusiasm," actual research is showing that we have up to a 3-hour anabolic window where muscle is prone to the uptake of protein and also that it is more important to have a "steady stream" of protein available during your recovery. My point? Eat or drink the protein. Ingest it regularly throughout the day keeping in mind your caloric needs/goals as well. Stop worrying so much about the anabolic window. Your gains are safe, bro.

Hydration

Drink plenty of water. One extremely reliable (and somewhat trivial) way to find out if you're hydrated or not is to look at the color of your pee. If you're adequately hydrated, it should be light yellow. For the sake of your social life, please never randomly share this information, but do take note of it. While we are here, you can adequately rehydrate post-workout by taking note of how much you weigh before you work out versus after your workout. Replace any lost weight with the same amount of water (i.e. if you lost 1.5 lbs, drink 1.5 lbs (~24oz) of water). It can be as simple as that. By the way, that Gatorade you're chugging right before a workout; it's mostly processed sugar. The electrolytes that it does provide really aren't necessary unless you plan to engage in intense exercise for more than an hour, or if you plan to exercise multiple times a day (i.e. you're a serious athlete). In any other case, you're pretty safe with just water. Any electrolytes you may have lost can be replaced via that super healthy and well-balanced diet!

If all else fails, my strong recommendation is to educate yourself and consult a nutritionist/dietician about your specific needs. Your diet is very, very important. But I urge you to dedicate most of your attention to the rest of the content areas in this book since this chapter was written by a very opinionated, border-line obnoxious exercise professional, and not dietician or a nutritionist.

6

Warm Up and "Stretch"

So, there you are. You've made it to the gym. If you are like many, many other people, you are looking at all the machines, all the equipment, the bands, the random things lying on the ground, and thinking to yourself, "Ahhh what the *&(#&#@! am I supposed to do?!" My recommendation? First, make sure you have read the rest of this book. That will minimize the occurrence of moments like the one described above. Then, warm up. Warm up first, always.

It has long been established that a good 5-10 min warm up is a great idea before jumping into a workout. However, many people get the warmup all wrong. This is not the time for static stretching (holding a position/stretching a muscle for more than a few seconds). This has actually been shown to increase the chances of injury during exercise and even decrease muscular strength/power. This is also not the time for jumping on a treadmill and slowly walking for 5-10 minutes; you probably already did that in the 30 minutes it took to prepare for and arrive at the gym. This is the time for dynamic stretching (moving your body/joints through full ranges of motion in a rhythmic and repetitive fashion) and a gradual increase in HR. Your goal is to elevate your body temperature, increase your HR well above resting levels, and to prime your muscles and nervous system for an impending increase in intensity. Nothing more, nothing less. It does not have to be extremely complicated. Your warmup can (and probably should) consist of similar movements that you perhaps plan to do during your workout. For instance, if you plan to squat with additional weight upon yourself (i.e. barbell back squat), you might elect to perform a few lighter, less-strenuous body weight squats as part of your warmup. If you plan to run, you may elect to perform some dynamic movements that mimic the biomechanics of running (i.e. butt kickers or high knees). These are just a couple of examples. Either way, take the warmup seriously, and I'll bet you have a better workout with a significantly decreased chance of injury. If you break a light sweat prior to your workout, you've done something right.

The issues I have with static/passive stretching:

People think it if you do it enough, it somehow elongates or lengthens muscle fibers permanently. This is not accurate. A lot of research simply shows that stretching allows our nervous system (the brain) to allow for greater ranges of motion. You must remember that all those muscle fibers are surrounded by nerves, blood vessels, and layer upon layer of connective tissue called "fascia" (I will talk more about this in Chapter 13). There are also tendons for each muscle and ligaments from bone to bone. All of that is surrounded by your skin. Imagine a sausage or brat inside its casing...inside yet another casing. Attach all of that to your bones with heavy-duty elastic tape. This is essentially how muscle is bound inside the body. Yanking on it repeatedly most likely would stretch out these connective tissues rather than the muscle fibers they encase. There are a lot of muscles. However, there is also a lot of fascia that most people seem to forget is there. I argue that all this stretching is not good for you for the sake of force transfer/production during movement.

Many people also believe that you should statically stretch after every workout because it helps with soreness and injury prevention. Nope. It doesn't. There is no consistent evidence that supports that consistent static stretching helps with soreness or injury prevention. As far as soreness goes, soreness is essentially caused by micro-tears (physical damage) within your muscle fibers. I can almost guarantee you that yanking on these tears will not magically repair them. What can? Proper recovery, nutrition, or perhaps even a light activity on your rest day that results in nutrient-rich blood flooding that area. And those things are not the result of magic.

In short, the industry trend is that people don't stretch enough. I suppose I am one of the few that believes people actually stretch too much. On top of that, we are stretching areas of the body that should not be stretched all that much (i.e. the hip joint). There are very few joints in the body built for stability; the hip being one of them. You go twisting and pulling on a stable joint too much and guess what? It becomes unstable, and instability is the enemy of strength and integrity. If you take a look at the basic human design from the perspective of an engineer, we are built to move fast and be relatively mobile. This makes us relatively weak beings. This is referred to in many texts as the "stability-mobility trade off." If a joint like the hip is built for stability, it is safe to assume it is not naturally very mobile. If a joint, take the shoulder, is built to be very mobile (we can move it through large ranges of motion in multiple planes), it is safe to assume it is not very stable. This is true. Due to this instability, the shoulder is extremely easy to dislocate. What about the hip joint(s)? Relatively much more difficult to dislocate. Without stability, you can have no strength. So... why are people electing to stretch every single joint they can possibly think of after every workout? Don't ask me. Because I really don't know. Does stretching have scientifically supported benefits? Yes. Am I saying never do it? No. I am saying we should start evaluating why we choose to engage in certain activities in the gym. I am saying that we should evaluate how much and what areas of our body we need to stretch, instead of just doing it because your gym buddy or Instagram trainer "X" said you should. I am not the first to offer the following perspective. I believe having too great of a range of motion and stretching too often can actually be harmful when trying to do anything athletic or move with any sense of stability/strength/structural integrity. As I mentioned before, muscle fiber and connective tissues have elastic properties. Thousands of people engage in plyometric training everyday due to this notion. We take advantage of these properties when we walk and run as a means of force transfer amongst our joints. During movement, this elasticity helps us absorb force and propel us in our intended direction. I offer that muscle and fascia can be likened to rubber bands. When rubber bands are brand new right out of the box, they do their job well. As long as they aren't over-stretched, they can grip things pretty tight, right? They develop tension well. When you over stretch rubber bands over and over, they either break or they become weak. They lose their elasticity and suddenly do not develop tension as well as they used to. I encourage you to not focus so much on stretching out your rubber bands and instead focus on activities that help their ability to effectively produce tension/force (i.e. strengthening).

Stretching has also been recommended for the sake of increasing mobility and/or flexibility. While I do believe these aspects of movement are very important, there should be a distinction between the two. I also believe one is more important than the other. Flexibility can also be referred to as passive mobility; this is how far you can take a joint through a certain range of motion with the use of an aid (like a band) or perhaps another person. In this case, you are trying to take a joint past its normal range of motion. This usually results in a moderate amount of discomfort. Mobility is more "active" range of motion is your "natural" range of motion that you can achieve under strictly muscular control. Raise a straight arm up over your head until you can't raise it any higher. This is your natural mobility. There's very little evidence that passive stretching increases mobility in the long term. Engaging in regular exercise can promote and even enhance mobility naturally. I believe mobility to be more important than overall flexibility. When it comes to stretching, my best advice is to consult a professional (physical therapist, skilled trainer, etc.) that can assess your structure/posture and point out the areas that need to be strengthened and the areas that need to be stretched/lengthened. You are working against yourself by stretching areas that need strengthening, and vice versa.

7

Aerobic vs. Anaerobic Exercise

Should we do aerobic exercise or anaerobic exercise? Cardio or weights? Which one is "better for me?" This might be one of the shortest chapters of the book. This is mainly due to the fact that I believe both forms are important for different reasons. My simple answer to these types of questions is I believe you should do both. There should be variation. A more complicated answer involves me saying "it depends" a lot. I feel I have already accomplished this; however, it definitely holds true here. Decide what your overall goals are and choose between them accordingly.

However, I will leave you with a few notes:

Continuous aerobic exercise has been shown to decrease overall muscle mass. The false words of many gym bros echo in my mind. They go around spraying the words "DoNT Do cArdiO cUz iT DestRYoys YoUR gAinZZzz BroOoOo." This is bunk. What they mean is, stay away from cardio like it is the Bubonic plague. It's all over if you raise your respiratory rate for more than 30 seconds. All of your resistance training goes to waste. No, this is wrong. The correct notion is you have to engage in a ton of cardiovascular exercise to affect your gains...bro. Going for a 2 to 3 mile run a couple times a week won't leave you looking like a twig. Consistently training for a marathon on the other hand...you get the point. Everyone will respond slightly differently.

Aerobic exercise is really, really good for you. In terms of increasing your chances of living a long, healthy life, it is arguably more important than resistance training. There is a much larger correlation between overall cardiovascular health and the prevalence of various disease states than there is between muscular strength/power and the same prevalence. One could argue the importance of bone health here, of course. However, please remember that I am a fan of both activities. There are benefits that each one provides that the other doesn't. There are reasons they are listed as vastly different activities. However, if I had to put all my money on one horse over the other in a race to live longer with better-overall health, I would put it on aerobic exercise. If there were a horse representing both, I'd find a way to borrow more money and double down.

There's a myth that floats around that low-intensity aerobic (relatively long-duration) exercise burns more fat than medium to high-intensity exercise. While this depends on many variables (weight status, fitness status, overall duration, etc.), this is generally not true. What people actually mean (whether they know it or not) is that low-intensity aerobic exercise burns a higher percentage of fat than medium to high-intensity exercise. Imagine a spectrum ranging from 0% to 100%. At any given time, your body is operating somewhere within that spectrum. The higher you go on that spectrum (the higher the intensity), the more your body is utilizing carbohydrates for energy. Additionally, the higher you go, the more calories you utilize per unit of time.

The complaint usually goes like this:

"I do a ton of low-intensity cardio. I am always walking. Why am I not losing weight/fat?"

First of all, if you have read every other part of this book, you'll know there is much more to the fat/weight loss equation. Some questions I might have for this person are:

- Are you getting enough rest?
- Are you stressed? *Important*
- Are you doing any other forms of exercise? If so, what? If not, why?
- What does your diet look like?
- Are you utilizing the FITT principle according to your specific needs/desires?

If you said yes to both questions 1 and 2, I would argue that your answer to question 1 was false. When I say rest, I really mean relief from all negative stimuli, both physically and mentally. If your brain is constantly in fight or flight, it ain't resting, which means the body is not adapting or recovering as well as it could. We will get to the brain and its ultimate importance in Chapter 9.

Let's say you had "perfect" answers to all of these questions. You are on top of your fitness game. There is still an issue here. The mistake most people make is thinking they are utilizing/burning more calories because they are utilizing more fat in this low intensity state. The key words here are "low" and "intensity". While you may utilize a higher percentage of fat within the spectrum, you are not utilizing more calories than if you were working harder for the same duration. Higher intensity exercise still utilizes fat. This is why high-intensity interval training (HIIT) has become more and more popular. It works. On top of that, while you may utilize a lower overall percentage of fat due to the intensity being so high (we use more carbohydrates to fuel exercise at higher intensities), it utilizes a greater *overall amount* of fat over the span of an entire workout. Let's say your 45-minute walking session utilized 300 kcal worth of fat. Okay, again. Let's say your 45-minute walking session utilized 300 kcal worth of fat. Theoretically, you can burn 300 kcal of fat in less time if you were working at a higher intensity. Also, it does not have to be a completely aerobic activity. Using weights is a great way to up that calorie/fat burn while keeping your workouts interesting. Don't make the mistake of thinking low-intensity exercise day-in and day-out is the magic answer to weight/fat loss. Throw in some progressive higher-intensity days and reap the benefits.

Note: Remember the individuality section of this book. Intensity is relative. There is nothing wrong with you if you need to start out by working at a lower intensity for a while. Just be sure to continue to challenge yourself or your body (and brain) will begin to shrug at your efforts (results will plateau).

Not only can weights be great for cardio, they are great for providing other beneficial stimuli for our bodies including mechanical and metabolic stress for our muscles, bones, tendons, ligaments, and other connective tissues. All become stronger overtime with consistent weight training. It is crucial that we include some resistance training in our programs, especially as we age.

8

BMI, Body Composition, and Body Type

Another common misconception many of us subscribe to is thinking the use of weights will cause a potentially unwanted increase in muscle mass (i.e. more weight). I'm here to tell you this is generally true. You will increase your muscle mass. But this does not necessarily mean you will have a dramatic increase in muscle size. On a side note, many females have a fear of bulking up with the use of weights. If you are a woman and this is your goal, bravo. Carry on. However, research has shown you have to be genetically blessed and consistently lift relatively very heavy to achieve such results. This includes a diet that promotes that result as well. The genetically blessed part of that will be discussed later in this chapter. For most women, it is extremely hard to achieve being "buff." Either way, fear not, having more muscle is a very good thing! More muscles cost more calories to maintain, thus a higher number of calories are utilized throughout your day. While this might result in an increase in the number you see on the scale, this should not alarm you. For it is not your overall weight, but your overall composition that really matters when it comes to health. What you are made of. Your fat-mass versus lean-mass. To put it even simpler, this is the amount of fat you have compared to the amount of muscle (and other fat-free things like organs and stuff) that you have. The goal should be to ultimately decrease your fat percentage and increase your muscle percentage, regardless of what your weight scale reads. Your diet should align with this endeavor as well.

There are a handful of pretty reliable ways to find out your body composition regardless of your location. In some places, they submerge you in a pool of water and see how much water volume you displace. There is also a giant egg-shaped container called a "Bod-Pod" that is widely available now too. Both have proven to be pretty dang accurate. However, if you simply want to get an idea or for the sake of convenience, many store-bought scales offer features that can "scan" your body for fat mass, muscle mass, hydration level and even bone mass. This is a technology known as "bioelectrical impedance." Basically, the scale/machine will send a very low-intensity electrical pulse through your body and scan for any "impedance" (blockage/interruption) along the way. The machine records the feedback and the more impedance it experiences, the more fat mass the scale reads. If this is your choice, just know the more hydrated you are, the more accurate your results will be. Many of us know that water conducts electricity quite well.

BMI

I am going to try and spend as little amount of your time in this section because of how unimportant this concept is. This stands for Body Mass Index and is found by dividing your body weight in kilograms (kg) by your height in meters squared. So, if you are 5'8" and weigh 220 lbs, you weigh 100kg (2.2kg/lb). There are 2.54 cm/inch. Take 68 inches multiplied by 2.54, that is roughly 172.7cm. Divide that by 100 (and round) and you get 1.73m. 100 divided by 1.73 squared (2.99) is about 33.3. That is your BMI score. Notice that it only takes into account your height and weight and doesn't take into account your body fat % or muscle mass. This means it is bunk. While this number can give you a general idea of your overall weight status, you should pay little attention to it. Overall body composition is by far more important. I have 11-12% body fat and more muscle than fat. I weigh 185lbs; I eat right and am a healthy weight for being

6'1". My BMI suggests I am nearly overweight; this is most likely due to my muscle mass. Anyone who tells you to make sure your BMI is in check has no idea what they are talking about. It is so unimportant that I wish it wasn't in my book and that you'd forget about it entirely. Let's move on.

Body Type

Around the middle of the 20th century, an American psychologist named William Sheldon came up with a theory that all people could be categorized into three main "somatotypes." You may have heard of the terms ectomorph, endomorph, and mesomorph. Each somatotype has their own structural (visual) and perceived personality characteristics. A lot of people might very well have characteristics from all three. It has become more and more popular to refer to these when people are discussing training protocols and diet strategies. There are many myths associated with this theory. Certainly, some people think it's more important for health, and others think it is bunk. While this is not my expertise, your body type might have an effect on its response to various diet and exercise habits However, I offer that the main "laws" of gaining/losing weight and muscle still and will always apply. To lose weight, you must be in a caloric deficit (more calories out than in). The opposite holds true if you wish to gain weight. If you wish to gain muscle, you must achieve progressive overload. If you happen to be aware of your body type and respond well to diets or exercise that favors it, then I say take advantage of that. If you have no idea what your body type is and have gotten desired results regardless, then I say...take advantage of that too. Do what works for you. Even if you don't subscribe to the Somatotype theory, do subscribe to the theory of a healthy diet and consistent, progressive overload. The key word being consistent.

9

Pain and The Brain

"He who treats the site of pain is forever lost." - *Karel Lewit*
"Where you think it is, it ain't." - *Ida Rolf*
"It is the victims who scream, not the criminals." - *Unknown*

I wanted at least one epigraph in the book, you found that included above. Including other people's quotes makes me sound like I know what I am talking about, right? I am sorry that I don't have cool quotes for every chapter. Anyways, this is the part where we return to talking about the brain. You may have gathered that from the chapter title…*Clears throat*. In my opinion, I think the book gets really juicy from here on out. Aside from the brain, other systems within the body are connected to each other via nerves as well. Let's talk about pain, the brain, and for the sake of our current century, texting. Wait, what? Just keep reading. Remember how I said the brain was the best security guard of all time? It is. It is the head security guard of your body. The CEO even. Other systems are its assistants or employees. If you're thinking slaves, seek help. Each system or employee has a different job that it is trained to do. When I use the word "system" here, I am simply referring to an organ, area of the body, or maybe a specific muscle or joint. System 1 reports a problem (pain) at its location in the "facility" (the body) via text (nerve signal). This is all fine except that system 1 did not send that pain report directly to the brain. System 1 told system 2 about it first. System 2 is overly confident in its abilities and decides to try and handle system 1's problem. It fails. Instead of letting the brain know, system 2 decides to forward the text that system 1 sent to system 3. System 3 also does not know how to handle this report and does the right thing and forwards the text to the brain. Here's the problem, the brain never leaves the office and the office (the skull) has no windows. Here's another problem, the brain receives this text from system 3, but there's no history of it ever coming from system 1 or 2. So, what does the brain think? There is a problem at system 3. It's wrong. Herein lies the point I would like to make. A lot of the time, the pain report will be forwarded by an organ or organ system that had nothing to do with the original source of pain or dysfunction. Your brain does not know the difference. All it knows is that there is a problem, but it has no idea where it originated. It just knows who sent the sad face emoji. What does this mean? Shoulder pain could mean ankle dysfunction. Hip pain could mean shoulder dysfunction. Neck pain could mean an issue with your breathing habits or the visual/vestibular systems. The brain doesn't actually know. It just knows something is wrong because that is the message it received. It is important that pain is assessed holistically. Structural issues and past injuries can in fact cause issues at the sight of the pain. A knee issue could very well be a knee issue. Just know that this perception of pain can spread to other areas of the body. It is important that we consider the body/person as a whole when dealing with pain.

Here is another funny thing about our brain's design. Our brain is divided into two separate (yet connected) sides or hemispheres. Most people know this part and leave it at that. However, it's important that we go deeper. Within the brain and spinal cord, there is a "crossover" of information. This essentially means we operate in an "X" shaped manner. What affects the left will affect the right and vice versa. What this actually means is that our entire body is also divided into two separate (yet connected) sides. Once again, an issue reported on one side of the facility might mean the origin of that issue actually lies somewhere within the opposite side of the facility. Woah! Yeah, there is a reason they have to text. Sometimes, it's not as easy as, God forbid, speaking face to face…

You might be thinking to yourself, "okay, so what do I do with this information? What do I do about my pain?" Well, there is no magical answer. I am just the (text) messenger. Do I expect you to now know exactly how to locate the source of all of your pain? Of course not. Once again, it is my hope that you simply become more aware after having read this book. It is my hope that the next time you experience pain in your shoulder or back, that you don't just elect to take some ibuprofen, or maybe massage that area and leave it be. Instead, I encourage you to think a little deeper and seek the help of a knowledgeable practitioner who can actually find and cure the problem at its source. Sure, a band-aid helps stop bleeding. But can it prevent further cuts? My issue is with thinking the solution to our health problems is the band-aid. The solution is at the source. The solution might lay within your daily habits. Take the proper steps to find the source! If I had to give you one answer to your pain, I would suggest you start to take the proper steps to cure it and prevent it. It is my hope that the entirety of this book will provide you with beginner steps you can take to prevent pain and injury before they occur. Sometimes the beginning steps to solving a problem simply come in the form of education and greater awareness. Pain, it's a call for change.

10

Squatting, Deadlifting, Power Lifts, Isolation, Etc.

If 4 people were reading this book at the same time, this is where I piss at least 3 of them right off. I put this topic last because it should be last. I know, I know. These have long been staples in both your and my workouts. The thing is that I don't really like em! The squat: the famous "king of all exercises." The deadlift: the king's polar-opposite twin brother who watches over the posterior side of the kingdom and plans to take the throne one day (maybe already has). The various power lifts: their distant, flamboyant cousins or something like that. This "royal family" rules over a kingdom of humans who bow down to their almighty will all day, every day, until their eventual demise at the hands of dysfunction, pain, and suffering. On the walls of various high school and college weight rooms read the names of humans who came and went, setting PR (personal record) after PR for these various movements. The royal family promises a life filled with structural integrity, athleticism, power, and strength. It's ingrained in our culture. I offer the notion that we are slaving away under the bar just to find the riches are short-lived. The gold, fake. The money, counterfeit.

Okay...it's probably not *that* bad. But for real, why all the hype? These lifts reign supreme. Yet, so does the prevalence of injury and pain in our society. Once again, this book is partly here to simply pose the question as to why this might be. Were our ancient ancestors in this much pain? Did they pick up and put down all this heavy crap all the time too? If so, it's a good thing they had the miracles of modern medicine, skilled surgeons/therapists, and knee braces to help them overcome all the aches and pains. Whew. Oh...wait, no they didn't. I am sorry but I don't think Julius Caesar was busting out 4 sets of power cleans in the back of the palace during his "me time." What was he doing during "me time?" Truth be told, I don't really know, and it's none of my business. That is between him and Mrs. Caesar. He was probably either sleeping or ruling a bada** kingdom. The point is, I don't think all these lifts helped him accomplish any of that. Nor were they popularized back then. You know what probably helped him though? Combat training (respects human function) and lots and lots of what you and I do every day but almost always take for granted: walking and running. We will get to that in a bit. First, kindly let me finish my rant!

Essentially, people are programming poor movement patterns into their brains and body through movements like hang cleans, deadlifts, squats, bench press, and other loaded bilateral movements that do not mimic the motor patterns associated with proper human functioning. I just don't think the brain likes it very much. Because the brain is wired for everything to work together in particular, predictable sequences, we experience pain and dysfunction when we "rewire" it by sending patterns it was not designed (by our DNA) to recognize. I am not saying I am 100% correct or that this is some proven theory. I am not saying people are wrong for squatting. But I am saying we should probably start paying more attention to this topic if we wish to experience less dysfunction and be in less pain. Pick your poison. If you are not getting paid (hopefully a great deal of money) to competitively squat, deadlift, powerlift, whatever...I highly suggest you reprioritize your training and the exercises you consistently perform. If your goals are to be as big and buff as you possibly can be, okay. Just know it will come with a high price later on.

It can be as simple as this true story about my brother and a shovel. When my brother and I were growing up, our parents had a house on a piece of 5-acre property. My brother and I were really into the *Lord of the Rings* when those movies were released. We would often role play, using random garden tools as weapons to fight off imaginary orcs (don't judge me). One day, my brother had a large shovel he was using to fight the invisible air orcs as if he were Gimli (the dwarf with the big axe). He repeatedly smashed the shovel into the side of the wooden animal pen that housed our goats behind the house. Mercilessly chopping away, he eventually broke the shovel. My stepdad was livid and bewildered how a 12-year-old could break a shovel. My brother was also confused how a shovel could break. After hearing the truth about what happened, my stepdad stated the obvious: "a shovel is not an axe dumba**!" My friends, the human body is not an axe. You cannot just use it against its intended purpose and expect it not to fall apart. Eventually, like that shovel, it will break.

If the topic of gait interests you, or you are thinking "I hate running, how can I train my body in a way that respects gait without always walking/running?" I suggest looking up the company "Functional Patterns" or even "DVRT." These are companies that are calling for a similar change in our training habits and I believe they just may be onto something big. Stay tuned for more evidence as to what I believe we should be doing in the gym instead.

In no way am I professionally associated with functional patterns or DVRT other than being your average social media follower. I do not claim to know their overall training methodologies.

11

Exercise and The Brain

So, what does the brain have to do with exercise? Well the short answer is everything. Let's take this topic by way of example though. When we are infants and start learning to walk, we suck at it. We have good intentions, but nonetheless, we fail. Over and over and over again. All this failure and sucking creates a high demand for adaptation within the brain. Your brain takes note of each detail associated with those failures. Then it sends out an adjusted motor signal, and we try again until the sensory feedback matches our intent. When our sensory feedback matches our intention of walking without falling on our face, the brain interprets this as success and stores that pattern for later use. So when the demand for adaptation is high, the brain responds by supplying that demand just as fast as it can. The same thing occurs when we do literally any physical activity that the brain has not yet experienced or perhaps has only experienced a few times. Certainly not enough times to prevent consistent failure. Not only does this apply to active movement, but also to static movement, such as posture. Your brain does not know any better. It can only interpret the input that is provided by your actions. If you are sitting with a rounded back, hunched over, staring at the computer (as I am doing right now, but this isn't about me, just keep reading) too often, your brain will receive and store this pattern. The more and more you send this nerve "pattern." the more it will interpret this posture as "normal."

Once again, what does this mean for exercise? Well, how you exercise matters. The movements you make and the form you take while executing movements matters. Too much exercise with poor form can result in pain and dysfunction. Remember, the brain does not know right from wrong. It just receives a pattern and stores it. The more it receives a particular pattern, the more it recognizes and labels that pattern as "normal." You might be wondering why can't the brain just adapt to this poor form, interpret it as "normal" and go on about its day? Well, the answer lies in what I believe to be our human blueprint. I believe there is a blueprint within our DNA that dictates how we are designed to move. If the demand for adaptation that you create for your brain is against our divine biomechanical purposes, we are left in pain and dysfunction. Again, I am not the only person on the planet that believes in this notion of a movement "blueprint." What is our divine biomechanical purpose? Locomotion. Moving from one place to another. Gait.

12

Gait (Walking/Running)

Here we are, human locomotion. Good ol' walking and running. Remember the first topic on individuality where I discussed universality versus variability? To remind you, this idea basically offers that we all develop similarly, yet individual differences exist. I believe this is not a coincidence when it comes to walking and running. I believe the reason all of us learn to walk and run is because we are supposed to. Our world requires movement from one place to another. We are designed for it, and our DNA and genetics ultimately dictate our design. I am not here to discuss any religious or philosophical topics. It is not my place to tell you how humans came about, or why we are here. However, it is safe to say that humans have been around for a really, really long time. Thousands of years. In that time, we learned to walk and eventually run. We transitioned from quadrupedal beings into bipedal ones. Why? The shortest and easiest answer is because it is more biomechanically and energy efficient. That is another great thing about the human brain and body. It favors efficiency. Even our minds are lured in by efficiency as we so often (for better or worse) choose to take the path of least resistance in our daily lives. I digress. It is safe to assume that given we (as a society) birth healthy children, they will one day walk and eventually run. As humans, we have been walking and running for thousands of years. Eager parents await the memorable day of their child's first steps. Walking is so common that almost all of us take it for granted each and every day.

Here is where the patterns come back into play. I know I pissed a few people off when I spoke about the (in)famous royal family of lifts. But, let me ask you this: On a day off of work, outside of the gym...how many times do you deadlift something relatively heavy on any given day? 2-3 times, maybe? How many times do you have hundreds of pounds upon your shoulders and squat with it there on any given day? I am going to guess zero here. How many times do you clean and snatch (pick something up and throw it over your head) during a given day or even week? Think about it. Maybe once when you fling a freshly laundered comforter onto your bed? Nice. This definitely warrants the use of a good, heavy clean and snatch in your workout program...not.

Let's shift in another direction. How many steps do you take each day? Even those who are minimally active may take well over a few thousand. I ran a half marathon a couple years ago where afterwards my watch read that I had taken roughly 49,000 steps. Wow. That is a lot of gait for one day. On a side note, I did not adequately prepare my body or brain for this half marathon, so gait became my worst enemy over the next few days. Anyways, sensory information (movement patterns) from each and every one of those 49,000 steps got sent to my brain during that half marathon. This happens thousands of times all day, every day. It's no wonder we begin to shrug at this activity. It becomes automatic. Besides, a lot of people don't enjoy going for walks/runs. I'll be honest, it's not my favorite. It's either torturous, boring, or both. So what happens? Those that don't like gait as a form of exercise engage in other forms of exercise that are more stimulating. This is all fine. Except for one thing. Many other forms of exercise (i.e. the previous chapter's content) and the methodologies associated with them go against the design of our biological blueprint. There are a great many practitioners (myself included) that are now blowing the whistle on this.

Gait is and always will be extremely important for humans. I'm telling you that it is what we are designed for.

How you walk/run can tell a skilled trainer/therapist a lot about any issues you may be having or any weaknesses that may be present within your structure. Observing gait is becoming more and more common in biomechanical assessment of human movement. There are a few potential problems that I want to mention that we definitely should remedy:

- A lot of people aren't walking/running enough, or they don't train at all (i.e. being sedentary)
- Other people do walk/run often, but don't train in the gym in a way that promotes and improves their gait (good motor patterns + bad motor patterns = suboptimal function)

- Other people hardly walk/run but DO consistently exercise, BUT they don't train in a way that promotes and improves their gait (ignoring gait + bad motor patterns = you need to read this book)
- A small number of people walk/run, and consistently train/lift in a way that promotes their divine function (Ideal, but currently not enough buy-in from the general population).

The first point above is just bad. The second and third are a bit better, but still not great. I think the point of greatness (fourth) is closer and easier to achieve than what most people think. We just have to be curious enough to discover it and patient enough to learn to do it.

13

Structure, Function, Tensegrity, and Fascia

Yes, that chapter title is written in English. One of the first concepts I learned about when I began my undergraduate studies was the idea that "structure dictates function." I imagine this an extremely important piece of information in many fields of work, but especially so in biology and kinesiology. "Structure dictates function" is to say that an organism's physical make-up will almost always determine how it functions, or in this case, how we move. Of course, this concept applies to the human body and every cell and tissue within it. Simple enough, right? Not quite. The problem I had with this concept is that after we learned it, we began to study each structure of the body in a somewhat isolated fashion. Unfortunately, this is much like how many people usually train their muscles in the gym. I suppose our educational journey was structured in this way to help promote learning about the body in intellectually accessible chunks. Unfortunately, it functioned to create a very fragmented, reductionistic idea of the human body inside of my mind and probably many of my classmates' minds as well. The notion that various physical structures of the body were connected and dependent upon one another nearly went right over my head. Unfortunately, I believe part of this was due to the severe lack of effort of a new adjunct professor (a physical therapist) that taught my functional anatomy course. I look back now and realize that I missed out on quite a bit of important information. I am somewhat ashamed to admit that it was not until during my graduate work that I began to consider every muscle, bone, tendon, ligament, and other systems of the body on a much larger and holistic scale. Then, a great many things regarding human anatomical structure and function started to make sense to me. It was an awakening of sorts. A series of "Eureka!" moments.

Given that our structure dictates our function, let's take a bit of a closer look at our mechanical structure. So for now, let's forget about things like organs, blood, skin, etc. I am referring mainly to the structure of our movement system: the joints, bones, tendons, ligaments, fascia, and muscles. The lever and pulley system of our body. I have found that not many people outside of this field think of the body in such a way. When we want to move, the brain sends a motor signal to the muscles it needs to recruit to accomplish the desired movement task. The muscles are attached to the bones via tendons. The motor signal reaches the muscle telling it to contract (shorten). This literal shortening of the muscle causes the tendon to pull upon the bone they are attached to. The limb/bone moves, and boom, we have movement. Movement is just a large, complex series of muscles pulling on bones in very precise sequences. Thinking about the body in this way allows us to see just how complex efficient walking and running is. On top of that, we become pretty good at walking and running by the age of 5 or 6. This is something that still amazes me every time I think about it.

Now let's consider the body's structure as a whole. Take a brief look at the full view of the entire body (front and back view) and all of the (superficial) muscles below:

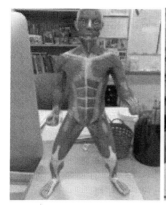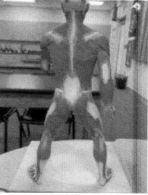

If we consider each joint, each muscle, and the attachment point of the muscle's tendons on each bone, we would quickly find out that the large majority of the body is made up of very inefficient levers. A wheelbarrow is an example of a very efficient lever system. You can place hundreds of pounds of material in the bin and along with the help of the attached wheel, relocate this material with relative ease. This is due to the very intentional placement of the fulcrum (the wheel), load (the bin), and relative length of the lever (the handles). There are only a handful of these types of efficient (strong) levers in the body. One example is at the ankle joints where our calf musculature meets our ankles. Most of us have the ability to quite easily stand on our "tippy toes" (referred to as ankle plantarflexion) and support our entire body weight for an extended period of time. We can even repeat this task over and over a great many times before tiring. Some of us can even do this on a single leg and hop up and down. This is an efficient lever in the body; one of only a few that is built for strength. Unfortunately, the great majority of all other joints in the human body are nowhere near as efficient as this. This goes to say we are relatively weak and unstable.

There is another concept in physics and kinesiology called the "stability-mobility trade off." This essentially states that there is an inverse relationship between a structure's stability and mobility at all times. If stability increases, mobility decreases. If a structure is built in such a way that it can freely move about (i.e. the shoulder joint) it greatly lacks stability. Thus, it is no surprise that the shoulder joint is one (if not the) most commonly injured joints in the body. Without stability, there can be no strength. Without strength, our joints do not handle large amounts of force very well. Herein lies the main point; given we are relatively unstable, mobile structures, we are not built for strength. So, what are we built for? What are we good at? Speed and mobility. We can move our structure at great speeds. Why do we need this? To accomplish efficient locomotion. Walking and running! It all goes back to that, folks. Don't believe me yet?

First let's go over the concept of "line of pull." Muscles develop force in the direction in which their individual fibers lay. There are few muscles that run almost entirely side to side (horizontal). There are more muscles that are oriented vertically (up and down) along our bones. There are an even greater number of muscles that are oriented in an oblique (diagonal) fashion upon our skeleton. A great majority of the muscles within the core are oriented in this fashion. Side note, the core is composed of over 30 muscles within both the upper and lower halves of the body. The core is not just your 6-pack abs or midsection. On yet another side note, that 6-pack is one of the least functional muscles within the core. The transverse abdominis and obliques are far more important. Unless your purpose is strictly to look better naked and your diet is beyond phenomenal, you can stop with all the crunches and leg lifts.

I digress. As I said, a large number of the major muscles inside the body are oriented in a diagonal direction. Given that muscles tug on bones, abide by their line of pull, and many of them orient diagonally, what does this mean?

We are physically built to rotate. Our anatomy favors rotation. Our bodies (and brains) love it. If you take a look inside any given gym at 5pm at night, you'll be hard pressed to find more than 1-2 people performing any type of rotational exercise. It's astonishing how many of us never break out of the sagittal (front to back) plane during a workout. Do you know what involves a great deal of the rotation our bodies crave? SURPRISE! Walking and running! As an honorable mention, I will include striking (punching, kicking, etc.) and throwing as well. You'll notice just about any powerful athletic movement involves rotation (kicking, throwing a football, swinging a baseball bat, swinging a tennis racquet, etc.) We are built to be phenomenal rotators, yet hardly anyone trains that way! I encourage you to remedy this trend.

Tensegrity

I am sorry but when you say a word like "tensegrity" people think you're at least 10% more interesting (nerdy). Try it out. There is a growing number of practitioners and educators who believe the body is structured as a tensegrity. If you are not sure what that is, don't worry, I have included a picture. The word tensegrity comes from the blending of the words tension and integrity. It is a term used in architecture and was coined by a theorist named Buckminster Fuller that described the eventual tensegrity structure created by a sculptor named Kenneth Snelson during the 1900s. This concept is actually quite common, and I am nowhere near the first person ever to suggest that the human body acts much like a tensegrity. There is even some evidence of tensegrity-esque structural behavior in biology at the cellular/microscopic level. Don't worry, we won't go that deep. Then you'd get the notion I was trying to convince you that I am some sort of smarty pants...

Anyways, I chose to include the topic in this book because I have never once seen this concept in my 6 years of formal education. Two degrees, a handful of professional certifications, and several seminars later, I have never seen it in a textbook or presentation. I felt this was extremely odd considering how very applicable it is to human structure and function. I could spend a few sentences trying to summarize this concept in my own words, but the Google definition should suffice. Google defines tensegrity as "the characteristic property of a stable three-dimensional structure consisting of members under tension that are contiguous and members under compression that are not." Translate this and apply it to the architecture of the functional human body, and you have the bones, muscles, tendons, ligaments, organs, and fascia (fascia will be discussed in just a bit). Basically, in a tensegrity you have solid structures suspended by non-solid structures that are balanced under tension. If the body is a tensegrity, the solid structures are our bones. The tensioned structures that suspend and ultimately help form what we know as the skeleton are our tendons, ligaments, muscles, and fascia. If you think about it, you'll realize that without the tensioned structures surrounding the bones and holding them in place, the skeleton would essentially fall into a pile of bones on the ground. A merry way to go about life, right?

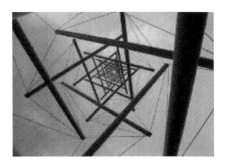

(A Snelson tensegrity structure)

Now, the interesting thing about a tensegrity is that when all of the "tensioned" structures are balanced, the structure is incredibly strong and able to withstand various forces placed upon it. However, each tensioned structure depends upon the relative tension and support of the next tensioned structure, and that one upon the next, and so on. Since every tensioned structure is dependent upon the next, if you were to lessen the tension upon one structure, it is quite possible that the whole structure would fail or collapse. I believe this is largely how the human body functions as well. Again, I will mention that it is extremely common that an ankle problem could eventually lead to a shoulder problem if left uncared for. Everything is connected by some means. Because everything is connected, every structure has the ability to affect every other structure, and this is crucial in understanding how you should go about maximizing your performance as a human being. Luckily, we aren't static and inanimate physical structures like Snelson's tensegrity. For better or worse, we are mobile and adaptable tensegrities. Thus, in order to move efficiently and without pain, we need to actively maintain structural integrity as we move about. Luckily, the brain does this for us as it receives an incredibly large amount of sensory feedback at all times from all parts of our body as well as our environment. A big shout out to all of our senses. Given the demands we place upon ourselves as we battle gravity, play sports, exercise and move about our world, maintaining our structural integrity while allowing for efficient movement is no easy task and there is a ton of room for a great number of structural failures. Another important characteristic of a tensegrity is that it always buckles at its weakest point. The human body is no different. On top of that, the human structure is quite lop-sided as it is. The odds of maintaining our naturally flawed structure in any way that does not result in pain are against us. Oh, and it just gets worse and worse as we age. Ahh, warms my soul.

Let's briefly talk about the brain again. The CEO. Both fortunately and unfortunately, the human brain has developed the amazing ability to assign the duties of one muscle to another when that muscle has failed or become injured. This occurs despite the fact that the newly assigned muscle was not designed or "trained" for that purpose. This is where the brain disobeys the rule that structure dictates function. The brain says, "well screw that, I dictate function." Thanks, brain. This allows the brain to get by for a while without totally closing for business ("collapsing" our structure). After all, the brain is all about efficiency and ultimately our survival. Eventually, however, that structure will send that dreaded text message. "Hey, I can't do this anymore. I want my old job back. Lol." And just like that, you are in pain. Tight muscles may very well be muscles that have been temporarily "reassigned" or even muscles that are relatively weak kinks in the armor. One or more areas of the tensegrity have failed, and it is now affecting your overall well-being. It is crucial that we change our ways when we exercise. It is imperative that we begin to train in ways that support our structural tensegrity. We can begin by ceasing to view (and train) the muscles, tendons, and other fascia as independent entities. It is important that our tensioned structures achieve "balance" and that this balance is consistently well-maintained to preserve our structure and ultimately our function. Again, I believe this begins and ends with optimizing your gait mechanics.

The Importance of Fascia

When was the last time you were in the gym or even talking to someone about exercise and you heard or used the word "fascia?" It has probably been some time. Or maybe never. I realize it is so rare that it is quite possible some readers might not even know how to pronounce such a word. I would bet that even if you are a certified trainer and you read that just now, that you thought "oh yeah, fascia. I remember...something...about that." While others may say it in various ways, I pronounce it "fa-sha" with a short "a" as in "apple." Fa-sha. Fascia. If that is wrong, sue me. Anyways, can we move on to what it is and what it does now?

Indeed, most people talk about either fat or muscle inside and outside of the gym. Rightfully so; they are trying to gain more of one and lose more of the other. So why am I talking about fascia? Because it is one of the most important pieces of the puzzle when it comes to movement. Even Leonardo Da Vinci included fascial-like details within his anatomical drawings. Although we are still not absolutely sure of its various functions in movement, the notion of its existence within us has been around for quite some time. So, what is it? Here, we can think of fascia as elastic connective tissue that connects various parts of the body (mainly muscles and soft tissues) to one another. This connective tissue provides a junction between various muscle groups. A lot of fascia also encases our muscles. Looking at your average anatomy text; you'd never tell as everything is presented in such isolated fashion. The fascia that encases muscle is known as the epimysium, perimysium, and endomysium. This fascia encases and organizes various groupings of muscle fibers. I liken it to sausage meat inside its fatty casing. Without it, the meat would not hold its convenient (and tasty), cylindrical shape. In order for our muscle fibers to efficiently create movement, they too must be bound and organized in similar fashion.

Brace yourself for one of the most important paragraphs in this book. There is even fascia that surrounds our *organs*. This "visceral" fascia responds to filling and/or inflammation of the organs. One of the most important nerves within the body is the "vagus" nerve, pronounced just like (Las) "Vegas". This nerve has several jobs including heart rate variability but is also responsible for sending status signals to the brain, letting it know how the organs are doing and if there are any potential issues. We can think of it as the AT&T or Verizon of the organs. Many, many text messages are sent via this service. Interestingly, the visceral fascia actually connects to the more superficial fascia. This fascia is more toward the "outer edge" of our bodies, within the muscles and bones under the skin. This is very important to understand. This means the status of our organs can affect our posture and resulting movement patterns, and vice versa.

Programming poor movement patterns in the brain can then affect just about every organ and system in your body. Poor organ health can cause much more than just a stomachache or fever. Could this be part of the reason exercise helps to eventually boost the immune system? Indeed, it assists in the maintenance and boosts the performance of all other systems in the body. Again, everything is connected in an extremely complex and purposeful manner. The brain receives a status report on everything at all times. It becomes easier and easier to see why what we put into our bodies and how we use our bodies (diet and exercise habits) are so intimately dependent upon one another. Exercise should be our daily medicine, not pills.

Let's get back to more of a movement-based discussion though. One of the most important superficial fascial tissues in the body is the "thoracolumbar fascia." "Thoraco" meaning the thoracic region of the spine/back and lumbar meaning the lumbar region of the spine/back. Aptly named, this fascia spans these two areas and connects two very important muscle groups together at the low-back: the latissimus dorsi (lat(s)) and the gluteal muscles (glutes). Two muscle groups that all the bros care so much about but almost never train them together. Why do the lats need this fascial connection with the glutes? The short answer is gait. The longer answer is that these two muscles work together to create stability at the hip during functional movement. Remember when I mentioned the "X" shaped neurological patterns we obey as humans? Here it is again. The left lat works with the right glute and vice versa. If you watch someone as they walk away from you, you'll notice that their left leg extends behind them at the same time their right arm swings behind them. Put another way, their left glute fires as their right lat fires. They work together and they are supposed to. This is not a coincidence that all able human beings share this gait trait (nice rhyme). This force transfer system is sometimes referred to as a "sling" or "functional line." The lat-glute connection is referred to as the Posterior-Oblique System/Sling. On the other side of the coin, if you watch someone as they walk towards you during this same instance, you will notice that their left arm swings in front of them as their right leg steps forward. Various muscles on the right side of the body fire with the right hip, once again to create stability as we move about. The left arm swings forward (the shoulder muscles cause this "flexion" of the arm) as the right hip swings forward (caused by the hip flexors). They are connected. This is called the Anterior-Oblique System/Sling. There are other slings and functional lines within our body as well, but these are two of the most important. If you have not already, can you begin to see why hip pain can mean shoulder pain and vice versa? Also, that the source of this pain may be on the opposite side of the body than which it is felt. Everything is connected. Pretty interesting (and sometimes sucky), right? Even more interesting is the fact that much of our fascia is elastic in nature. It captures force/energy and transfers it elsewhere much like a rubber band does when you pull it back and flick it across the room, or perhaps at the back of someone's head. Recall that I mentioned our muscles rubber band-like nature earlier when I bashed the concept of mindless stretching. This elastic property is largely due to the presence of fascia. I know what you must be thinking. "Wait, so we are just big hormone-filled lopsided rubber-bandy tensegrities with brains that often fail us?" Yes. Exactly.

Now, imagine you are walking in slow motion. The right heel strikes the ground. The force created between the ground and the heel strike (ground-reaction force) is absorbed by the leg muscles, joints, bones, and fascia and then "ripples" up and around the body via more and more fascia. The thoracolumbar fascia intercepts some of this force and redistributes it along the opposite side of the body where more fascia will intercept and transfer it. Eventually, some of this ground-reaction force reaches our jawbone as I mentioned earlier in this text. Now speed it up. Think about walking, or better yet, get up and walk 10 steps and think about all of the force being developed by the muscles at work, absorbed by the various structures (both tensioned and not), and transferred throughout your entire body with every given step. It's quite amazing how we just develop, absorb, and transfer force in various directions. The product of all of this is the resultant movement throughout our environment. Let's remember we are simply talking about going for a nice stroll. Think of sprinting, kicking a ball, or making a swift change of direction while playing football. The body can successfully and repeatedly withstand all of these forces. Amazingly, we can make all of these seemingly violent movements look graceful and smooth.

Our bodies are intricately and purposefully built. It is not as random as it may seem. My point in mentioning fascia is that it serves an extremely important role in the elastic harnessing/transfer of forces throughout the body, across the tensegrity. Many of the common movements we see in the gym these days do not properly utilize our fascial network, let alone, in a functional manner. This movement includes slow speed isolatory exercises as well as the "royal family" of compound lifts I mentioned earlier. Attempting to train our muscles in isolation goes against our amazing design and ultimate purpose. All of the stressors, injuries, and dysfunctional movements our body compensates for every day can eventually lead to weaknesses within our tensegrity. To properly recruit all of this fascial tissue, we have to attempt to utilize the entire body in a way that respects our innate structural design. This is how I would define "functional" training. If an exercise or program does not promote truly "human" function, I do not see how it can be considered functional. I believe the word "functional" to be one of the all-time most misused terms in the exercise industry. To explore even more on fascia and functional slings/lines, I suggest looking up Tom Myers (who also studied with Buckminster Fuller, the creator of the tensegrity model) and his concept of Anatomy Trains. His work has greatly inspired my writing and practice. See also Andry Vleeming and Dianne Lee's work on Slings. I mention them here to highlight their potential importance now and in the future of exercise.

These ideas might seem novel to some. You might be thinking "Gee, this makes sense." Google these terms and you will find there are several (free) sources available allowing all of us to explore these topics. Once again, it has been around for a long time and seems to have been nearly forgotten about within our current "reductionist" framework for viewing the human body. The information is out there. My intent in mentioning these concepts here is in the hopes that you won't ever forget how important it is in our biomechanical functioning. I encourage you to find ways to exercise in a non-isolated, holistic fashion that promotes the preservation of your tensegrity. I cannot stress the importance of this enough.

14

Tips for Training with Respect to Human Design

Are you wondering where to start? I sure did when I came across all of this. Luckily, I have some answers for you. If you are like me and walking or running aren't your first choices, here are some guidelines for resistance training:

1) Perform movements that mimic the biomechanical patterns (limb movements) of walking/running. Recreate the muscular contractions and joint motions as closely as you can, whenever you can. Start with the shoulder and hips or arms and legs. As we know, when one side of the body flexes, the opposite side extends. We are unilateral beings. The two sides of our body work independently, yet they are very well and meaningfully connected. Take advantage of that.

2) Rotate. Rotate. Rotate. Stop performing/prioritizing so many bilateral movements that move your joints in one plane/direction. Prioritize unilateral exercises in the transverse (rotational) plane. (If you need further explanation here, please look up the three main planes of motion associated with human movement) I will talk more in depth about this in the following chapter.

3) Perform more ballistic/explosive movements with respect to walking/running mechanics and the fascial lines.

Exercises/movements that use the functional lines:

Gait (Anterior and Posterior-Oblique Slings) and the Lateral Line: Walking and running, of course. Skater Bounds with arms driving the side to side movement. (Imagine the motion of an ice skater sprinting to top speed) Running in place. Skipping.

Superficial Back Line: Jumping Medicine ball (MB) slams, Battle Rope Slams, Superman holds, Box Jumps

Superficial Front Line: Jumping MB slams, Battle Rope Slams, MB Chest Passes, Hollow Holds, Box Jumps

Spiral Line: Cable chops from various angles, hitting a punching bag, unilateral cable presses/pulls, throwing a frisbee, and hitting a forehand/backhand in tennis.

If you are not trying to attack gait mechanics directly, try and simultaneously activate muscles that work well together, such as the lats and glutes, or the pecs (chest) and contralateral (opposite side) obliques. This will create neurological connections and solidify functional movement pattern within your brain. Take 15-20 minutes and look up the "functional lines" of the human body. Explore new and interesting ways to move.

It should now be no surprise that I offer the following statement. Walking and running are two of the best forms of assessment for judging your overall quality of movement. While I am not the biggest fan of treadmills*, having someone film you from multiple angles (preferably in slow-motion) as you walk or run on one can give you an idea of how you look as you move. I suggest eliciting the help of a skilled practitioner so they can also help you see where there may be areas of weakness within your structure based on your gait cycle. This can give you some good insight as to what you should then prioritize when you train.

Remember, it all comes back to the sensory feedback patterns that your brain is receiving. If you give it poor/conflicting patterns that are not in accordance with your body's design, you will have poor adaptation and eventually poor structure/function. The more you tell your brain what is important, the better it adapts. I posit that it adapts best to what it knows best: gait patterns. Lastly, you should tell your brain what is best often. Very often. The greater number of overall stimuli you create, the quicker your brain adapts. I liken it to memorizing a song that you like. Hearing the song once doesn't do much for the brain. But listening to a song you like on multiple occasions over several days or weeks provides a great neurological stimulus and demand for memorization. Send those sweet melodies to the brain enough, and it can recall those auditory patterns for years to come. Movement works the same way. Consistently provide your brain with functional stimuli. Make sure the frequency of that stimuli is adequate for long-term adaptation.

I don't feel that treadmills provide us with a truly realistic running experience as the ground beneath you is constantly moving backwards. Every time your foot lands, it is shoved back behind you regardless of your intent. This can possibly cause or exacerbate knee pain and other lower extremity pain. I always suggest to clients that run consistently that they try and run outside on real ground (preferably softer ground like grass). Spending some time outside in the sun is good for you too!

15

Rotation and Unilateral Exercises

I would like to thank and credit Andreas Saltas for the inspiration to compose the following chapter. Andreas Saltas is a New York-based physical therapist known on social media as the "Bodmechanic." I believe him to be one of the best and most honest practitioners in the business and highly recommend you throw him a follow on Instagram.

We are lopsided. We are not symmetrical, and we never will be. So many people in the gym (especially body builders) train for symmetry. While some might achieve, or come very close to achieving visual symmetry, humans will never be truly symmetrical from a physiological or biomechanical standpoint. As far as I know, there are two main reasons for this. One, we are built lopsided. And two, our brains usually always favor one side of the body (usually the right). Meaning our neurology is asymmetrical as well. There is one organization that even bases their entire methodology on this principle. Look up "Postural Restoration Institute" to learn more about their methodology and therapeutic approach.

If we vertically bisected our body into two halves, and then placed each half on a separate scale, we would find that the right side of our body actually weighs a bit more than the left. This is due to the placement of the organs (mainly the liver) and a couple extra lobes of tissue within our diaphragm and our right lung. All of this causes a postural phenomenon that is essentially out of our conscious control. In many cases, the rib cage will compensate by rotating and "flaring" out to the left side of the body. This causes compensatory movement in other areas of the body. The rib cage almost reacts like an accordion. Since the left side is now flared, the right side of the rib cage follows left, but also "collapses" the accordion on that side. This can actually be seen with the trained eye. The brain is aware that this rotation occurs, and many times will cause the hips to rotate to the right to counterbalance the left-rotated rib cage. Now, we are probably talking millimeters of movement here. However, over the span of years and years of moving on and within this "twisted" structure, this can make quite the difference in our movement patterns. I mention it here to suggest that we should probably move away from doing so many heavily loaded bilateral (strengthens/activates both sides of the body simultaneously) movements such as the squat or deadlift for example.

Let's take a look at the squat for a second. While I mentioned that it is hard to judge other people's movements because of variability, I think we can level here and say that some squats just look terrible. Whether there is inward (medial) knee collapse on one or both sides, twisting or rotation of the body as we descend/ascend, or others., all sorts of compensatory patterns are possible. It may be partly due to the fact that we are trying to perform "balanced" movement upon an imbalanced structure. Now, this may be due to much more than just a rotated rib cage or pelvis. I believe part of the solution lies in reprioritizing our exercise choices and performing more unilateral movements and perhaps even performing more work on the left side of the body. Indeed, any endeavor toward postural symmetry requires an asymmetrical approach. This is another reason I believe many of our answers lie within optimizing gait, the most efficient and natural unilateral human movement pattern.

16

Posture and a Foot Fetish

It's a working title. Bare with me. Many people think posture has a lot to do with the position of your shoulders/upper back. Are you slouched? Are you often bent over at a desk? You must have bad posture then. So, what do we see and hear everywhere? "Sit up straight," "retract your shoulder blades," "don't round your back; it's bad for you!" This really isn't how it works. Like, at all. Wouldn't it just be wonderful if postural manipulation was that easy? Unfortunately, it is not. Your resulting posture, while it may show up in your shoulders, actually begins with your feet. Of course, it is also very much connected with and affected by the state of your brain. Remember that any structural manipulations must first be approved by the brain. At any given moment, your posture is the product of the overall state of your tensegrity. Which parts are tight? Which parts are loose/weak? Is there balance? Why are they tight/weak? Can we remove or lessen the stimuli causing this? Do we need the addition of other stimuli to get us where we need to be? We must remember that while we are a dynamic and adaptable organism, we are very much a mechanical structure that operates upon the principles of physics. After all, muscles are really nothing more than ropes attached to "solid" structures (bones) that pull them in the direction most oriented with the direction that their fibers lay. We are a system of pulleys and levers.

Any and all adaptations to our structure are based upon overall demand. More importantly, it is the frequency of that demand that matters. The demand for adaptation is either created by us and/or our environment. Sitting in a chair for 8 hours with rounded shoulders and flexed hips for one day is probably not a bad thing. Sitting in a chair for 8 hours, for many days throughout your life definitely is a bad thing. Especially if you are inactive otherwise. Rounding your shoulders or back is not bad for you. It is something our structure very much allows for and is necessary for various movement tasks. However, adapting to a posture featuring rounded shoulders and flexed hips is not ideal. This adaptation can only occur through a consistently imposed demand. Create a stimulus, expose the body and brain to it enough, and you will get adaptation. The important question is, is the stimulus you are exposing your structure to resulting in desirable adaptation? Is it a state that leaves you in minimal/no pain? Is it a state that can comfortably withstand the demands of everyday life? What stimulus are you giving your structure and how often? Obviously, this is where the importance of exercise lies: to give our bodies the necessary stimulus for desirable adaptation. One of the biggest problems here is (as previously discussed), most people think that any and all exercise is good exercise. Hopefully, you have a better idea now that the specific demand (the exercise/movements you engage in on a regular basis) matters equally as much as any other aspect of the FITT principle. Consider it a subdivision of "type." Now, where do the feet come in? My answer to that is, of course, at the bottom of the legs...That was a joke and I suggest we move on before I lose you.

The feet are extremely important members of our structure. They are like one of the best friends of the brain. If the brain ever got to step away from being CEO for a few days, it would most likely spend its free time playing video games and getting drunk with the feet and their roommates (the ankles). Continuing to childishly personify, the amount of attention the brain pays to the feet would be, in any social situation, unsettling to most third parties. Luckily, the feet love it and will probably never file a restraining order. The feet are needy and require a great deal of care and the brain is there to provide. The brain showers the feet and ankles with (literally) billions of gifts in the form of nerve endings. The feet return the favor by providing the brain with lots and lots of sensory information coming from the ground (our body's only consistent contact point with the earth beneath us). Given that we are bipedal beings, it makes a lot of sense that the brain would require a great deal of info coming from down there. Here is the thing. If the feet are weak or structurally unsound, then that affects everything all the way up the structure. When the feet call out for help, whether they like it or not, the brain relies upon the rest of the body to help. Unfortunately, like I discussed previously, they are the worst friends, and they suck at helping.

Given a consistent stimulus and enough time to do so, the structure adapts all the way up. The result of any and all adaption (good or bad) is our posture. If the feet are unhappy, so are their roommates (the ankle). Here is another reminder that everything is connected. Positioning at the ankle affects the knee, which affects the hips, which affects the spine, which affects the rib cage, which affects the shoulder blades that sit upon the rib cage, which affects the neck, and boom: we have posture. And remember, I am not just referring to the bones and joints but the muscles and fascia too! Consistently poor stimuli results in tightness here and weakness there, all the way up the chain. If you're lucky, you might achieve balance in various places. So, long (and socially unacceptable) story short, take care of your feet. Strengthen them. A shoulder problem may be a knee problem, which may be an ankle problem to begin with. Check on the feet first. Don't look to blame the bad friends, look for the original whiner and help them to suck it up and realize life sucks, but it's okay because there is cake. Mmm, cake. Let's move on.

Tips:

If your job or lifestyle currently dictates that you sit for most of your day:

- Get up and walk around for a few minutes every 15-20 min if you can. This will help with blood circulation amongst other issues associated with chronic sitting. Walking also provides the body with "natural" stretching and joint mobility. This is especially beneficial for your feetsies.

- Fidget. Twitch. Bounce your knees up and down. Move and adjust your posture often. Remind your brain that it's wired for movement. 1 hour in the gym a day is hardly enough. That leaves ~15 hours (not including sleep) of room for error, every day. Move often.

- Hydrate. Always adequately hydrate.

- If you wear shoes, try not to. Shoes are the a**hole ex-lovers of your feet (assuming your feet are capable of dating). They are the relationship your feet never wanted but still has to put up with because you shop at the same stores. Gross. Shoes make our feet weak. I can almost guarantee you that many of your foot-related complaints are due to the unwanted wearing of shoes. Have a low arch? You don't need inserts or orthotics, you need strength. You need increased sensory input from your feet. When our feet are introduced to support, they tend to start depending upon it. This makes them weak and passive structures. Orthotics and the like are another bad friend and exist because people in podiatry want to make more money.

- If you must wear shoes, I highly recommend investing in barefoot/minimalist shoes and wearing them whenever you can (remember, frequency). This can also help give your feet that strengthening they desperately need. "Vivobarefoot" is my shoe of choice and they offer many styles for both recreational and professional needs. Their CEO poses the question, "when you get home from a long day at work, what do you do? Kick your shoes off." The body and brain seem to prefer this state.

17

Training as You Age

It is unfortunately inevitable that we all age and eventually expire. While there is no stopping this process, it has been shown that regular exercise can significantly slow it down and preserve our function. No matter your age, I believe the entirety of this book applies to how you should go about exercising. It's never too late to start a journey toward better function. Now, I don't know what it is like to be 50-60+ years old. However, I have worked with many people who are in that age range. Aside from general aches and pains, both my experience and a lot of research has shown that the aging population is ridden with various pains and diseases such as back pain, knee pain, osteoporosis, and arthritis. It is fair to say that many of my clients have had jobs that required them to be somewhat sedentary. Certainly, this will become more of an issue in the future as technology continues to allow the workforce to sit on their bums. In a way, it is nice that many of us can be relaxed at the workplace. However, it only makes sense that I would be mostly unsupportive of this trend. Physically, it is hurting more than helping us. You might think then that I'd be all for standing desks. Nope. I don't believe we should stand in one place for 8-10 hours a day either, letting gravity have its way with compressing our already very compressed, dehydrated joints. A happy medium is necessary. Getting up and moving around often is necessary (doing so outside if possible). Getting our heads out of our phones and taking a look around us more often. Providing our brain with healthy stimuli is basically the only way to avoid random chronic pains.

Given the prevalence and risks of osteoporosis as we age, it makes sense that resistance training should definitely be a part of the equation. Consistent and progressive mechanical stress upon the bones and outlying structures (tendons, ligaments, muscles, fascia) creates the stimulus needed for the body to lay down more bone tissue, more muscle, more fascia. Once again, this does not just mean picking up heavy things and putting them down in any way you please. The specific sensory input you provide for your brain and whether that agrees with our innate structure and function matters a great deal. Your resistance training should be intentional. Here is another reason I offer that running/walking are the king of all exercises for the human body. They stress all systems and structures simultaneously.

Another common issue the aging population face is that of balance and the risk of falling. Indeed, most of the older clients I have worked with have had poor balance. This is a multifactorial issue involving the nervous, muscular, visual, and vestibular systems. If your vision is poor (and uncorrected via lenses), your balance is likely poor. Again, the visual and vestibular systems are anatomical neighbors and work well with one another. If your balance is poor, certainly, you may run the risk of falling. Should you tip one way or the other, it is now the job of the nervous system to send various signals to your muscles in an effort to stop yourself from falling. Almost automatically, the brain will tell your legs and arms to act in such a way to increase your overall base of support. This reaction can even be seen in infants as young as 4-6 months (parachute reflex). These actions require a great deal of coordination and strength. Not only that, but one often overlooked aspect in exercise regimens within this population is power. Power is how much force you can develop per unit of time. Another term for it is "speed strength." Many older people have the strength to hold themselves up if you slowly tip them onto one leg. However, do they have the power to create that strength fast enough should there ever be a need? And believe me, if you're about to fall on your face, you best hope there is some amount of power available within you. Many people (including a lot of trainers) seem to think that the elderly population is too frail for power training. I call BS. Perhaps when they are just beginning an exercise regimen, they are. However, this does not mean they should never move quickly. Just like strength, power is relative. Sure, they are not going to crush a baseball like Barry Bonds. However, the elderly should move as powerfully as they can, and they should do so often.

Important notes: Training with power is considered high intensity and is more stressful upon the human structure than say, endurance training. Higher velocities are involved. Care should be taken that you have been training at a lower intensity for a significant period of time before introducing a significant increase in powerful movements. Training with maximal power too early can be unsafe. Power training also features lighter weights compared to strength or endurance training. Oftentimes, power training can be accomplished using no weight at all (using your body weight). The goal here is really to train the nervous system, not so much the muscular or skeletal systems. Another benefit is that powerful movements often recruit more/different muscle fibers and can make for a really well-rounded exercise stimulus. I am not saying power training is all you should ever do. But it should be introduced at some point and then consistently included as you age.

18

Core Training

Aside from the word "functional," the word "core" is probably the second most misused term in the industry (maybe even the world). Despite the ever-popular belief, the core is not just your abs or midsection, and the crunch is possibly one of the worst and least functional exercises of all time. Depending on how specific you want to be, there are over 30 muscles within the core. A better and still fairly simple way to think about what comprises the core is this: the core is all tissues that stabilize or act upon the spine and hips. Given that definition, things become a bit more complicated. I am not going to get into what I think are the best core training exercises (because most are isolatory, aka junk). I will say this, training the core is highly important. It is hard to move with any sort of quality if these muscles are not coordinated and strong enough to handle the task at hand (whatever that might be). Since I won't mention any isolatory exercises, what then do I leave you with? I leave you with a suggestion; that you refer back to the end of chapter 14 on "training with respect to human design." I believe the core is designed to stabilize our bodies to allow for efficient transfer force throughout our structure. To say it a different way, I believe the job of these muscles is to stabilize our center of mass so that the outlying structures (the arms and legs) can move with increased leverage as we navigate our environment. Certainly, without core strength we could not efficiently and powerfully throw a ball or move a large piece of furniture, for example. Strength cannot exist without the presence of precise stabilization and leverage.

Many of the muscles within the core are designed to work intimately with one another. Our overall design is based on total-body movement through gait. Train accordingly. Train your gait mechanics with respect to your tensegrity-esque structure and you can be sure the core is being trained too. There is no functional need for thousands of crunches or 3-minute planks. Activation of the core musculature is largely dependent on breathing mechanics as well. There is a reason breathing out (exhaling) during exertion is recommended. A forceful exhalation will help activate (amongst others) the transversus abdominus, one of the most important spinal/core stabilizers. Another important aspect of breathing is the activation and use of the external and internal intercostals (the muscles between your ribs). A mobile rib cage is very crucial when it comes to accomplishing sound posture and functional rotation of the upper body. It starts with skilled breathing. I cannot overstate the importance of being good at breathing. And I'm not referring to belly breathing. I mean breathing that moves and expands the rib cage (more on this in a bit). This is where posture (not referring to sitting upright, but an overall healthy balance amongst your tensile structures) becomes increasingly important. A posture that locks down the rib cage in a dysfunctional position will alter your breathing performance. Altering your breathing performance could have significant effects upon your cardiovascular system, which then have an effect upon (but not limited to) muscle, nervous system performance, and even various organ functions. The list goes on. Everything is connected to everything, so everything affects everything!

19

The Lymphatic System

I dedicate this chapter to my late uncle, John, who lost his 9-year battle with a rare form of bladder cancer in February 2019. I cannot imagine the inner strength it took for both my aunt and my uncle to take on cancer together for nearly a decade. The day I wrote this passage, it had been exactly one year since his passing. I would also like to thank my mother and dedicate this chapter to her work as well. My mom is a certified lymphedema therapist and an expert in the lymphatic system. She has positively made a difference in the lives of hundreds of cancer survivors, including my uncle's before his passing. Without her, I would have never been inspired to write, and I may have never found out just how important the lymphatic system is for each and every one of us.

The lymphatic system is hands down the most under-appreciated, underrated, underserved, and under respected system inside the human body. Here are a few important aspects of the lymphatic system:

> 1)   It is part of the venous (return) system. The lymphatic vessels run almost parallel to that of the major veins throughout our bodies. As most of us know, veins bring blood back toward the heart. Wherever there is a vein or venule (smaller vein), you can assume a lymphatic vessel is close by.

> 2)   It is responsible for carrying all of the excess protein-rich fluid that our vascular system doesn't have room for. Indeed, our veins overflow at times, depending on a host of factors, including blood

pressure. This excess fluid that cannot be held by the veins is then picked up (absorbed) by the lymphatic vessels where it eventually gets dumped back into venous circulation near the heart. Meaning it, once again, becomes part of our blood. While it is traversing the body inside the lymph vessels, the fluid is known as "lymph fluid" or simply, "lymph." Most of us know that every cell in our body comes into contact with blood and its contents all day, every day. This obviously means that every cell comes into contact with lymph fluid then too. Cells are constantly undergoing maintenance. Substances go in the cell, and substances come out. All day. Every day. The lymphatic system is there to help intercept some of those substances. Big whoop, right? Keep reading.

3)   Aside from the vessels that carry around all this lymph fluid, the lymphatic system contains over 600 bean-shaped structures called "lymph nodes" that are interspersed throughout the body. Most of them reside from the mid-chest, in the armpits, groin and on upward toward the head/neck. A great many are located around the base of the neck. As lymph travels through, these lymph nodes act as "filters" that house various white blood cells that are responsible for detecting and eliminating bacteria, antigens, and some viruses within the fluid. These lymph nodes are essentially a very important extension of our immune system.

4)   The lymphatic system is also responsible for the transport of large molecules that are too big to make their way through normal vascular circulation. This can include the transport of large fat molecules. Fat.

Something many health-minded individuals, like you and I, are very much concerned with. Hmm…possibly important? I think so.

Lymph Movement

There are only a few ways to effectively move lymph. Breathing, movement, or manual therapy, like what my mom does. Let me tell you, there are not many of her around. Certified Lymphedema Therapists are harder to find than functional exercises done in a public gym. There are roughly 2100 LANA (Lymphology Association of North America) certified therapists in the US. Most of which are in the medical field: physical therapists, occupational therapists, and massage therapists helping those with lymphedema-related issues. They have no time to be concerned with your lack of movement. And no, you cannot have my mom. What does this tell you? First, if you don't breathe efficiently, your lymphatic system is probably suffering. Second, if you don't move well and often, your lymphatic system is probably suffering. Third, I am a momma's boy and am not ashamed.

So why aren't we concerned with the lymphatic system then? In my entire 6 years of formal education, I believe this system was mentioned one time. Then, I, and I'm sure every other student in the lecture hall, forgot about it. I'm here to stress to you: DON'T forget about it. It's an intricate system that runs parallel to and is intimately connected with our arteries and veins. It's one of the MVPs in our body's overall immune response. It takes care of large fat molecules and makes sure they go where they need to in order to be stored (or hopefully, metabolized). Without it, you'd cease to exist. It sounds like it's very much on our side, no? Dr. Perry Nickelston, author of *Stop Chasing Pain,* is a New Jersey-based, world-renowned health practitioner and chiropractor. He offers a lot of great information on the lymphatic system on both Instagram, his website, and in his course "Lymphatic

Mojo." I highly recommend checking his work out. He describes the lymphatic system as the filter to our body's "aquarium." When an aquarium doesn't have a properly functioning filtration system, the water becomes murky, and bad things might happen to little Nemo (our cells). When our cells are constantly exposed to a toxic, murky environment filled with their own waste, they certainly don't function optimally. Then, we start to feel like poo, and we wonder why. *Big thumbs down*.

Our lymphatic system is prone to becoming murky. It's prone to becoming backed up, or "clogged." You can bet that when your lymphatic system is compromised, all other systems will be compromised as well. What causes all this? Well, lack of movement, sucky breathing, and poor diet just to name a few big ones. We should all be aware that there are some cases where the lymphatic system can become compromised or altered against one's will, even if they are succeeding at the above-mentioned lifestyle aspects. There are genetically influenced lymphatic disorders (i.e. lipolymphedema) that affect only females. There are also many cases where surgical removal/alteration of lymph nodes can affect an individual's lymphatic system for the rest of their lives, leaving them prone to lymphedema (i.e. cancer survivors). It is important these individuals find consistent and reliable treatment. Since I have claimed sole rights to my mother, what can the rest of the human population possibly do? There is hope. So, what are the only other options to move lymph and keep this system clog-free? Breathe well, move often, and eat right. Sounds just about as easy as everything else in the book, right?

Super Sucky Stucky

Say that five times fast. My friends, it's important we breathe well. Not only so we don't pass out and die, but so

we can also keep our lymphatic system happy too. I know what you might be thinking. "Isn't breathing at all technically breathing well?" Unfortunately, no. It is very common to hold the stresses of life within the musculature of our shoulders and neck. I am confident that if you are an adult with a job and responsibilities, you have definitely felt this before. When this happens, our neck and shoulder muscles eventually become overactive (tight) in trying to help us breathe. Lack of movement and poor posture cause our rib cage to become "stuck" and immobile. Thus, breathing becomes sucky. Super sucky. Super sucky stucky. Get it?

In a perfect world, the neck and shoulder muscles mind their own business, do their own job, and our diaphragm and intercostals (muscles between the ribs) do the great majority of that breath work. Again, in this perfect world, there'd be a lot more people like my mother running around too. Unfortunately, this just isn't the case. I cannot overstate that rib cage mobility and use of the rib cage when breathing is extremely important. Anyone that tells you to "belly breathe" clearly has ulterior motives and should get a new mother; one more like mine. Okay, I'm just kidding (kind of). Anyways, learn how to breathe and practice breathing well. Be mindful of it. It helps with way more than just your lymphatic system. What about moving often? Proceed to the final chapter.

20

Putting It All Together

Variation, Volume, and the Zones of Movement

There is somewhat of a paradox created between the introduction of a stimulus to the brain/body and then manipulating or changing that stimulus. How often should that change take place? Many different health and fitness professionals will offer various answers. I think it depends a lot on your personal intentions. The more important question is if and why should you change that stimulus. If a movement (or lack thereof) causes you consistent or chronic pain, this most likely means your brain disapproves of that stimulus. A change should probably occur.

Now, there are many movements that the human body can perform. Obviously, here you have come across a few that I definitely approve and disapprove of. Again, it seems to me that there are a few fundamental truths about human movement that will always hold true. Gait, rotation, consistent positive stress (aka eustress), practicing high-quality rest, adequate nutrient intake, and so on. These are all aspects that, when the quality of each is maximized, I would deem being within the "safe zone" of the overall human experience in terms of health and movement. There are many things that do not fall in this safe zone, and instead enter what I will trivially call the "danger zone." Certainly, these zones will vary from person to person. At that, we are really talking about poor movement patterns and/or extreme "volume." Here, I refer to volume as simply the overall number of stimuli the brain

receives with little regard for the quality of that volume. Too much or too little of any stimulus can be detrimental to the body. While not necessarily detrimental, even too much stimuli within the safe zone can halt progress. This might sound increasingly complex (it is), but don't let me lose you just yet. We are almost at the end of the book for crying out loud.

There is no one successful protocol that holds true for everyone. We all have different genetics, experiences, and histories. We all have different genetic potential and developmental tendencies (refer back to chapter 1 on "We are all the same at being different"). This is why I believe variation in your exercise is absolutely necessary. Certainly, too little movement or variation can lead to a poor or weak stimulus for adaptation. Thus, little progress occurs within the brain and body. Let's say for example that it was proven that lunges were overall the single most beneficial exercise for all human beings. If all I ever did was perform lunges in the same environment, at the same time of day, in the same exact way, at the same speed, every single day of my life, my brain would essentially get bored and no matter how good those lunges were for me, adaptation would cease. Thanks, brain. It is important we change it up, but also that we don't leave the safe zone too often, and definitely not for good. The problem with many exercisers is they often vary their exercises/routines, but they do so by entering and popping up a tent in the danger zone. Yikes.

Second to that, yet equally as important, is volume. This is how much overall stimuli (stress) your brain and body are experiencing on a consistent basis. Low movement volume (i.e. sitting around and reading health books too much...) leads to zero demand for any type of positive adaptation and possibly, should you ever need to move with any sort of integrity, it leads to an increased chance of injury due to weakness, tightness, lack of coordination, visual and vestibular problems, pain, etc. Too much of too little can

cause injury, pain, discomfort, illness, you name it. Finding a happy medium is important. The same goes for the overall "volume of variation." The question being, how often and how much are you varying? The brain loves new stimuli and change. It loves something new and different to chew on. However, it is important that these changes are tactical (they serve a purpose), gradual, structural, and functional. It is important we vary our activities all while residing in the safe zone. I believe if we take the time to craft our own individualized exercise/lifestyle recipes, the safe zone becomes quite large. The more you move, the larger your safe zone becomes. Let's dive more into this in the following sections.

Environment

Throughout the world, modern gyms are one of the most popular locations to exercise. We construct large buildings which house various exercise equipment that provide us with many different movement options. The gyms then invite the masses to come experience that for a monthly fee. It is extremely convenient and a great money maker; it is certainly a great business opportunity. However, many people purchase those memberships and hardly ever use them. I often wonder why that is. For one, gym owners bank on this. Certainly, people have a slew of reasons as to why they don't make it to the gym all that often. I feel one of the most important, though, is the overall environment. Here, I will leave you with another crucial piece of information. Sensory input drives motor output. Read that again. *Sensory input drives motor output.*

Gyms are often crowded, dimly lit, loud, and indoors. I don't believe this naturally bodes well for a healthy environmental stimulus. It's really no wonder why many people would rather stay home. While daily trips to the gym are a smart decision, we should vary the environment in

which we choose to consistently exercise. Or should I say, we should vary the environment in which we choose to exercise consistently. Either way, what I mean is to go outside sometimes. Too much sun is obviously bad for most of us. A little every day is very good. Being outside in open areas also allows for the eyes and other sensory systems to explore movement outside the confines of a crowded gym floor. Go to the park, a beach (if you can), or a nearby mountain trail. In addition to your gym trips, perform different types of movements/activities outside and vary it often. The brain loves this variation and for lack of a better phrase, it keeps us young. Consistently poor-quality sensory input received by the brain (i.e. info from all senses, poor diet, movement patterns, and environment) will cause poor-quality motor output.

Let's say you own a nice car with a supercharged V8 engine. This thing is beautiful and fast, and it's the only one you will ever have. It requires premium fuel and the finest oil to operate at its best. Would you go and put regular unleaded fuel with dirt and Fruity Pebbles mixed in inside your gas tank? Probably not. Yet, many of us seem to readily do that to ourselves. Our own bodies! Our brains (our once in a lifetime supercharged V8 engines) require that premium fuel and oil too. This comes in more forms than just enough carbs and adequate sleep. High-quality and adequate nutrient intake is essential to fuel it, but high-quality movement and sufficient rest is the oil that keeps that baby running smooth. And that V8 needs a fill-up and a couple quarts every single day.

Challenge All Systems

I have discussed many of the important body systems that are usually stressed during exercise. The cardiovascular

system, the muscular system, the nervous system, and so on. While these are important, they often eclipse the importance of challenging and stimulating the other systems that have a massive influence upon pain and the overall health status of the body. These include the vestibular system, the visual system, the fascial system, the lymphatic system, and specific "branches" of the nervous system such as the parasympathetic and sympathetic branches of the nervous system. Other than a bunch of large words, what am I really saying? Roll around, jump, run, bound, bounce, skip, hop, summersault, look all around you, play catch, get up and down from the ground, creep, and crawl. Do things you are bad at. Play. Experiment. "Did he just tell me to act and play like a little kid?" Yes. Definitely. Both kids and adults are straying from these activities that used to be natural for us as we grew up, and I believe it is a mistake. Perform movements that challenge all systems simultaneously and the function of these systems will be maintained and enhanced. Do all of this while you...

Respect the Human Body

Remember our innate structure and function as previously discussed. It matters. Move accordingly and move often. Don't do too much too soon. Make consistent progress using the FITT principle as a starting point. Rotate more. Integrate all systems and parts of the body. Get outside and walk more. Lift weights. Change it up. In such a stressful world, make the effort to find out what activities or environments put you at ease; move in those environments. You owe it to yourself to rest well and often. Put it all together and life starts to feel pretty darn good. Wash, rinse, vary, repeat.

Now please, put this book down and go move.

Although, I highly recommend you refer back often…

Okay, go. But remember…*exercise is bad for you.*

ABOUT THE AUTHOR

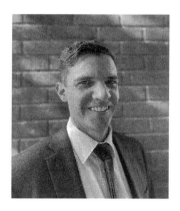

Tyler Thoms, 27, was born and raised in the Bakersfield, CA area. At the age of 11, his family relocated to Tehachapi, CA. Tyler attended Tehachapi High School from 2006-2010 where he became the school's most decorated tennis player of all time. After graduation, Tyler attended both Bakersfield College, and California State University, Bakersfield, during his undergraduate work; eventually changing his major from Communications to Kinesiology.

In 2016, he graduated from CSUB at the top of his class with a Bachelor of Science in Physical Education and Kinesiology. Shortly after becoming an NSCA Certified

Strength & Conditioning Specialist, he opened his own personal training practice, privately contracting and gaining experience at several gym facilities around the Bakersfield area. Somehow always involved in sport, he also became an avid golfer around this time. In late 2017, he began an accelerated online graduate program through California University of Pennsylvania, graduating magna cum laude a year later with a Master of Science in Exercise Science and Health Promotion.

In the summer of 2019, he became the head varsity tennis coach at Bakersfield Christian High School. He also became an adjunct professor at CSUB where he still teaches kinesiology coursework to undergraduate students. Tyler has plans to open a non-profit business for the benefit of youth athletic programs in Kern County, CA.